...Devices

Other books in the Essential Clinical Skills for Nurses series

Monitoring the Critically Ill Patient
P. Jevon & B. Ewens
0 632 05803 X
978 0632 05803 7

Intravenous Therapy
T. Finlay
0 632 06451 X
978 0632 06451 9

Pressure Area Care
K. Ousey
1 4051 1225 5
978 14051 1225 3

Respiratory Care
C. Francis
1 4051 1717 6
978 14051 1717 3

ECGs for Nurses
P. Jevon
0 632 05802 1
978 0632 05802 0

Practical Resuscitation
P. Moule & J. Albarran
1 4051 1668 4
978 14051 1668 8

Stoma Care
T. Porrett and A. McGrath
1 4051 1407 X
978 14051 1407 3

Care of the Neurological Patient
H. Iggulden
1 4051 1716 8
978 14051 1716 6

Central Venous Access Devices

Care
and
Management

Lisa Dougherty
RN, RM, Onc Cert, MSc
Nurse Consultant
Intravenous Therapy
The Royal Marsden NHS Foundation Trust

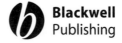

Blackwell
Publishing

Editorial offices:

Blackwell Publishing Ltd, 9600 Garsington Road, Oxford OX4 2DQ, UK
  Tel: +44 (0)1865 776868
Blackwell Publishing Inc., 350 Main Street, Malden, MA 02148-5020, USA
  Tel: +1 781 388 8250
Blackwell Publishing Asia Pty Ltd, 550 Swanston Street, Carlton, Victoria
3053, Australia
  Tel: +61 (0)3 8359 1011

First published 2006 by Blackwell Publishing Ltd

ISBN-10: 1-4051-1952-7
ISBN-13: 978-1-4051-1952-8

Library of Congress Cataloging-in-Publication Data

Dougherty, Lisa.
Central venous access devices : care and management/Lisa Dougherty.
      p. ; cm.
  Includes bibliographical references and index.
  ISBN-13: 978-1-4051-1952-8 (alk. paper)
  ISBN-10: 1-4051-1952-7 (alk. paper)
  1. Intravenous catheterization.   2. Blood-vessels –
Cutdown.   3. Nursing. [DNLM: 1. Catheterization, Central Venous –
nursing.   2. Catheterization, Central Venous methods.   3. Catheters,
Indwelling. WY 100 D732c 2005]   I. Title.

  RC683.5.I5D68 2005
  617′.05 – dc22
  2005016454

A catalogue record for this title is available from the British Library

Set in 9 on 11 pt Palatino
by SNP Best-set Typesetter Ltd., Hong Kong
Printed and bound in India
by Replika Press Pvt Ltd, Kundli

The publisher's policy is to use permanent paper from mills that operate
a sustainable forestry policy, and which has been manufactured from
pulp processed using acid-free and elementary chlorine-free practices.
Furthermore, the publisher ensures that the text paper and cover board
used have met acceptable environmental accreditation standards.

For further information on Blackwell Publishing, visit our website:
www.blackwellpublishing.com

Contents

Foreword

This book provides a long overdue but invaluable resource for all healthcare practitioners involved in the management of central venous access devices (CVADs). It contains a wealth of up to date, evidence-based information that is essential if high quality care and minimal complications are to be avoided during the patient's intravenous (IV) journey.

Each chapter provides essential information regarding the technical aspects of clinical assessment, the insertion of each device and the signs and symptoms of problems that may occur, pre- and post-insertion. Irrespective of individual devices, the author adopts a highly sensitive style throughout when considering the effect having a device placed and subsequent therapy may have on patients' lives.

The central venous system is not only important for the critical management of many patients in anaesthesia and acute medicine but a crucial pathway for intravenous therapy. The number of patients requiring central venous access continues to grow as the management of oncology, dialysis, trauma and infection improves, and life expectancy is prolonged. The result is an increasing population of patients who require reliable venous access over long periods of time. CVADs are literally lifelines for patients in a wide array of circumstances, and therefore maintaining reliable and safe vascular access is the prime objective of this book to aid healthcare workers involved in the delivery of intravenous therapy via the central venous route.

This book provides reassuring advice for healthcare workers involved with CVADs in the acute setting and those who may not have immediate access to experts in this field. Increasingly important are the legal and professional aspects of patient care, which are discussed within the text, together with suggestions on how to best inform patients about living with a CVAD.

The introduction to this book provides a helpful overview of the venous anatomy with informative text regarding each vein that contributes to the central venous system. Particularly helpful is the detail afforded to the general features of CVADs, their design, length and diameter, aiding the reader to appreciate the effect this can have on veins housing a device. Within the introduction, clarification is given regarding the correct position of CVADs within the central venous system, an important but controversial issue amongst some healthcare disciplines. This section eliminates any misconceptions, describing each element of a CVAD in detail and providing comprehensive evidence to support clinical practice.

Catheter materials and design are discussed in language easily understandable to those unfamiliar with the subject. With so many products now available the choice cannot only be overwhelming, but costly. Factors influencing CVAD choice are discussed and include issues such as finance, lifestyle and the effect a device may have on a patient receiving IV therapy in a community setting. Emphasis is placed on patient assessment, clinical condition, device selection, intravenous therapies and the experience of the operator. This text encourages healthcare workers to consider the potential therapies patients may require, not just their immediate needs.

Gaining IV access has historically been somewhat of a chore for junior doctors and so the discussion regarding specialist IV teams, who systematically include clinical assessment, venous and device selection, patient positioning, relevance of anatomy and physiology in preparation to insert a CVAD, is a useful aide memoire for operators and assistants alike. The detail afforded to the procedure itself is practical and informative.

The second chapter deals with the subject of peripherally inserted central catheters (PICCs), devices increasingly used in organisations throughout the world for various IV therapies. The practicalities of PICC insertion, the risks and benefits are all well explained, with a useful scenario towards the end of the chapter describing complications that can occur with PICCs.

The following three chapters discuss non-tunnelled, short-term CVADs, skin-tunnelled CVADs and implanted ports. In each section the recommended use for each device is discussed, and scenarios relating to the device are included at the end of each chapter. The chapter on subcutaneous ports is highly informative, with emphasis once again placed on selecting the right device for each patient. Risks and benefits plus complications found uniquely in the use of ports are discussed within this section.

In Chapter 7 the author highlights the fact that, unfortunately, nature is not always kind: the venous system is extremely variable and even where anatomy is reasonably constant there is considerable risk of injury to vital structures during the insertion of a CVAD, unless precautions are taken. The serious complications associated with the removal of a CVAD are also discussed.

In Chapter 8 the comprehensive practical management of complications associated with CVADs is extremely well illustrated and provides an excellent and systematic approach to problem solving, with key suggestions to avoid recurrence. A useful table is included which summarises recommendations from the main organisations for the management of complications. Emphasis is placed on the high risk nature of CVADs in the hands of inexperienced personnel and the book stresses the importance of continuity in a simple step-by-step approach if serious complications are to be avoided.

Throughout this book the patient's perspective is never forgotten, including practical issues regarding mobility, social issues and the importance of education and training.

The aim of this book, to inform healthcare workers of the fundamental principles associated with CVADs, has been achieved. It takes the reader from an introduction to central venous access, through advanced practical clinical assessment and insertion of CVADs, to recognition and management of technical complications. This comprehensive, well referenced, evidence-based text brings together all the elements in an elegant and systematic manner. It is an essential resource for all healthcare workers involved in the management of patients requiring central venous access.

Helen Hamilton
Senior Nurse Specialist in Vascular Access
Oxford Radcliffe Hospital NHS Trust
RGN, BSc (Hons), FRCN

Preface

Central venous access devices (CVADs) can be utilised for most types of intravenous therapy and provide reliable venous access for long-term access or immediate access in the emergency situation. In the past, CVADs were used exclusively in specialist hospital settings such as critical care and oncology. However, now, with the development of new catheter technology, easier and safer insertion techniques and improved selection for patients, CVADs are used in a variety of areas in both acute and community settings.

The first chapter provides an overview of the main types of CVADs, their advantages and disadvantages. A key feature of this chapter is the importance of patient assessment (which includes choice of vein). It examines anatomy and physiology in relation to the insertion of devices, and properties of the catheter (diameter, length, material and design) in relation to selection of the device. This chapter also contains a section related to whom should be inserting devices and this is particularly relevant as an illustration of the expanding role of the nurse. Specific issues related to the environment, skin cleaning, position of patient, use of ultrasound and anaesthetic, diagnosis of tip placement and documentation are also covered.

The subsequent chapters consider the four main types of CVADs: PICCS, non-tunnelled central venous catheters, skin-tunnelled catheters and implanted ports. Within each of these chapters the devices are defined and described, and the indications for use, advantages and disadvantages, insertion, immediate and follow-up care and removal are all provided, along with the relevant practical procedures. The chapter on management of CVADs covers the importance of securing and dressing a CVAD, the rationale for maintaining patency, the importance of site inspection and methods for taking blood samples.

Chapter 7 covers the hazards of insertion, listing the signs and symptoms of the most common complications and the prevention and management of each one, such as pneumothorax, air embolism and catheter malposition. Chapter 8 provides the management of complications once the CVAD is in situ, as 15% of patients who undergo central venous catheterisation have complications. Nurses have an important role in detecting and treating them promptly to reduce their effect and, wherever possible, to prevent them. These include catheter damage, infection, thrombosis and extravasation.

Finally, Chapter 9 presents the patient perspective to provide readers with an understanding of the issues related to living with a CVAD and how it can impact on a patient's life. It provides discussion of the educational needs and some practical advice on developing information materials. The appendix provide sources of information, such as Royal College of Nurses Intravenous Forum, Infusion Nurses Society (INS) and Association of Vascular Access (AVA), as well as key textbooks.

The aim of this book is to provide an overview of the central venous access devices for both those who wish to gain new knowledge and understanding related to caring for these devices, through to the more experienced nurse who wants to explore the text to provide evidence and support for their practice. The book does not provide information on certain types of catheters that are used in more specific areas, such as haemodynamic monitoring and dialysis catheters, but rather it aims to provide the fundamental knowledge required to care for and manage the more common CVADs, whether in the hospital or community setting.

Lisa Dougherty

Introduction

Central venous access devices (CVADs) have been in use for many years and they have been referred to in the literature and by healthcare professionals as 'long lines', 'central lines', 'Hickman lines' and 'port a caths'. This chapter aims to introduce the reader to the terminology, types and general aspects of CVAD insertion.

LEARNING OBJECTIVES
By the end of this chapter the reader will be able to:

(1) Define a CVAD.
(2) List the main types available.
(3) List the advantages and disadvantages of using a CVAD.
(4) Discuss the requirements of patient assessment.
(5) Understand the relevant anatomy and physiology associated with CVAD placement.
(6) List properties of central venous catheters.
(7) Describe the relevant issues related to insertion.
(8) Discuss the issues related to consent.

DEFINITION
A central venous access device is a device whose tip lies within the lower third of the vena cava (superior or inferior) or the right atrium (Stacey et al. 1991; Davidson & Al-Mufti 1997; Royer 2001; Galloway & Bodenham 2004). The device itself may:

- start in a peripheral vein (as in a peripherally inserted central catheter or PICC);
- be directly inserted into a central vein (non-tunnelled central venous catheter);
- be tunnelled under the skin (skin-tunnelled catheter);
- be implanted (implanted port).

Terminology

'Long line', Hickman® line (Bard) and Portacath® (Sims Smiths Industries) are either trade names used by the companies, or slang, and can be used by practitioners to mean different things. For example, a 'long line' may be used to describe a PICC, but the tip may only be located in the subclavian, which is not a PICC and could confuse the user.

The medical definition of a central venous access device is one whose catheter tip lies in the thoracic vena cava. Midline and midclavicular have been referred to as 'long lines', 'halfway midlines', 'PICCs' and 'extended peripherals'. Midline and midclavicular have been mistakenly called PICCs. PIC has been used for peripherally inserted catheter, rather than a central catheter, leading to confusion, and which could have serious ramifications (such as an extravasation injury), if inappropriate solutions or medications are infused via these devices when they are placed non-centrally (i.e. the tip not in a central vein) (NAVAN 1998).

Therefore it is important that generic terms are used wherever possible in everyday use and the author has provided the generic descriptions for the different devices.

Standardisation of terminology for these devices should be limited to:

- Peripherally inserted central catheter (PICC): where the tip is located in the lower third of the superior vena cava (SVC) (NAVAN 1998; INS 2000; RCN 2003).
- Midline: where the tip is located in the upper arm, not in a central vein (Perucca 2001; RCN 2003).
- Midclavicular: where the tip lies distal to SVC, i.e. innominate, subclavian or axillary veins. The placement of a catheter tip in the subclavian is also known as midclavicular, and may be preferred for delivery of therapies with low potential for vein irritation. A concern is the decreased vessel size, curvature and flow velocity in the subclavian, which may be a factor for the increased risk of thrombolisation in these catheters. It is also difficult to know where the tip ends from the outside, unless it is clearly identified (Goodwin & Carlson 1993; Carlson 1999).

• Skin-tunnelled catheters, non-tunnelled catheters and the catheter attached to an implanted port: all these devices have their catheter tip in the vena cava or right atrium.

USES

CVADs can be utilised for most types of intravenous therapy, but there are some specific reasons why a CVAD would be chosen instead of a peripheral intravenous access device:

(1) To provide reliable venous access for patients requiring long-term access (for parenteral nutrition, chemotherapy, etc.).
(2) To provide immediate access in emergency situations or post-surgery, for rapid infusions of fluid, blood or blood products.
(3) To monitor central venous pressure.
(4) To provide venous access for patients who have poor peripheral venous access.
(5) Patient choice.

ADVANTAGES AND DISADVANTAGES

The main advantages and disadvantages for using a central venous access device can be found in Table 1.1.

Table 1.1 Advantages and disadvantages of a CVAD.

Advantages	Disadvantages
• Provides reliable long-term access.	• Increases the risk of infection.
• Able to be used to take multiple blood samples.	• Increases the risk of thrombosis.
• Can be used to administer blood, blood products, medications, nutrition and fluids.	• Subjects the patient to risks during insertion, such as pneumothorax, haemorrhage.
• Removes the need for constant venepuncture and/or peripheral cannulations.	• Can be a traumatic procedure for patient to undergo.
• Can be used to monitor central venous pressure.	• In some case it may require a general anaesthetic for insertion.
	• Can affect body image.

OVERVIEW OF CVADs

Whilst each chapter is dedicated to explaining each type of device in greater detail, Table 1.2 provide a quick overview of the main types of CVADs currently available.

PATIENT ASSESSMENT

Ideally, the patients should be involved in the decision as to which CVAD would be most suited to their lifestyle and therapy, although patients requiring central venous access post-surgery and in an emergency situation may not be involved. However, all patients will be assessed for the best type of device, the safest location and which offers the least risks (see Table 1.3). The following aspects should be assessed, usually by the practitioner inserting the device, but any nurse caring for the patient is still able to assess certain aspects that will help both practitioner and patient to select the most suitable CVAD.

Patient's diagnosis

Certain groups of patients with a specific diagnosis may have recommendations made regarding their venous access by expert groups. For example, the Clinical Haematology Task Force (1997) made the following recommendations for all haematology patients: that tunnelled catheters should be used, single lumen are preferred but multi-lumen catheters may be used for specific indications, and that ports are more suitable in children.

Venous anatomy

In spite of the vast numbers of veins in the human body only a few are considered suitable for a central venous access. The main veins used include the internal jugular, subclavian, axillary and femoral veins. A systematic approach to the selection of vascular access sites and planning of future placements can reduce risk of unnecessary venous stenosis and scarring.

Concurrent medical conditions

Table 1.4 gives the conditions that should be considered when deciding which catheter is best suited to each individual patient.

Table 1.2 Overview of CVADs.

Type of device	Material	Veins commonly used	Design	Number of lumens	Insertion requirements	Dwell time	Associated complications
Peripherally inserted central catheter	Polyurethane Silicone	Basilic Cephalic Median Cubital	Open-ended Valved	Single or double	Good antecubital access unless ultrasound used	Months up to a year	Phlebitis Infection Thrombosis Malposition Occlusion
Non-tunnelled central venous catheter	Polyurethane May be coated with antiseptics; antimicrobials or impregnated with silver ions	Internal jugular Subclavian Femoral	Open-ended	Single, double, triple, quad or quin	May require ultrasound if jugular route used	10–14 days	Occlusion Infection Thrombosis Pneumothorax
Skin-tunnelled catheter	Polyurethane Silicone	Internal jugular Subclavian Femoral	Open-ended Valved	Single, double and triple		Months to years	Infection Thrombosis Occlusion
Implanted port	Portal body – titanium or plastic Catheter – silicone	Internal jugular Subclavian Femoral	Open-ended	Single or double	Ability to undergo GA	Months to years	Infection Thrombosis Twiddlers syndrome Extravasation

Table 1.3 Assessment for the selection of an appropriate device.

- Type, rate and duration of treatment (vesicant/irritant properties; osmolarity/pH).
- Patient's personal requirements and ability to manage self care.
- Environment and social influences.
- Variation in equipment.
- Availability of skilled practitioners to place device.
- Skill and experience of carers involved in day-to-day management of patient's CVAD.
- Suitability of target vessels.
- Co-morbid conditions.
- Numbers of concurrent and intermittent infusions (e.g. compatibility).

(Egan Sansivero 1998; Jackson 2003)

Therapy requirements

The duration of the therapy may impact on the type of device suitable. For example, a PICC would be suitable for 4–6 weeks of treatment, but a tunnelled catheter would be more suited for therapy of six months or longer (Cole 1999). If the patient were to receive multiple therapies that are incompatible, a single lumen device would be unsuitable. Viscous solutions may require a larger diameter device, which may exclude some PICCs.

Lifestyle and quality of life issues

Patient choice is a major consideration. Patients need to understand the degree of care required for each device, their appearance after placement and any restrictions on their level of activity. Consideration should be given to the dexterity of the patient, as well as the type of physical activities that the patient may undertake, e.g. use of crutches, driving and the discomfort of a seat belt, and the continuation with sporting activities. Issues surrounding small children and pets and the possible risk of dislodgement should also be considered, along with any implication regarding intimacy and sexual activity for the patient (Hamilton 2000). For example, physical activity can increase the risk of phlebitis and dislodgement. It may also be more difficult to conceal a PICC from public view (Cole 1999). A port can promote feelings of well-being because it provides the patient with privacy about their physical status.

Table 1.4 Issues related to medical conditions.

Medical problem	Issues
Orthopaedic problems	May limit access in upper limbs due to deformities as a result of arthritis or surgery. May affect the patient's ability to lay flat or gain access to veins, e.g. kyphosis.
Malignant disease (solid or haematological)	Patients with solid tumours are more likely to develop thrombosis, and disease that has affected the upper lobes of lung, trachea or oesophagus may cause difficulties on insertion and increased risk of complications. Haematology patients may demonstrate abnormal clotting profiles and therefore have more potential for bleeding. Previous treatments, such as radiotherapy, can cause localised tissue to become altered in density and texture in patients who have undergone these treatments, and the position of veins may be distorted.
Septicaemia	Patients with septicaemia are more likely to be clinically unstable: tachycardic, hypotensive, tachyopnoeic, which could result in problems during insertion.
Inflammatory bowel disease	Patients with chronic conditions such as Crohn's disease usually require long-term parenteral nutrition, and repeated insertion of CVADs can result in stenosis and increased risk of associated thrombotic complication.
Infective endocarditis	Patients often have deposits of infected plaques adhering to the valves of the heart and therefore there is a risk of displacing these and causing further contamination when inserting CVAD.
Renal disease	Patients are at greater risk of thrombosis as well as the need for careful site selection to preserve veins for future use.
Severe epilepsy	May displace device during a convulsion or cause difficulties during insertion, resulting in complications.

(Hamilton 2000)

Table 1.5 Factors influencing CVAD choice.

- Risk of infection
- Physiological issues
- Frequency of accessing
- Duration of treatment
- Convenience of CVAD in relation to activities of daily living
- Number of complications associated with CVAD
- Type and amount of care required
- Location of placement
- Availability of a caregiver
- Body image

(Adapted from Chernecky et al. 2002)

Patient involvement also encourages greater compliance with care and it appears from the literature that patient satisfaction outcomes are higher (Cole 1999) (see Chapter 9 for more details). Chernecky et al. (2002) listed characteristics that are considered important by patients and intravenous nurses when choosing a VAD (see Table 1.5) and highlighted that choice of a CVAD is a collaborative process involving patients, carers, the practitioner inserting the device, nurse and doctor (Egan Sansivero 1998).

Current condition of the patient
Table 1.6 gives the functions and status of the patient that may influence the type and location of the CVAD.

Ability to position patient as required
It may be necessary for a patient to be placed in positions that may be difficult or may not be suitable, depending on the patient's condition, such as tilting the head during the procedure. This can be problematic for patients with respiratory problems. During the insertion of a PICC the patient may be asked to turn their head to the side of the insertion and move their arm so it is important that these movements are checked prior to insertion. If the patient is unable to change position it may make the procedure more difficult and put the patient at a greater risk of complication, such as malposition.

Table 1.6 Current conditions to be considered.

Clinical status	Considerations
Haematological stability	There should be agreed parameters of the clotting profile, platelets etc. and the reduction and cessation of any anticoagulant therapy, to ensure that haemostasis will occur, in order to minimise the risk of haemorrhage during insertion. It may be necessary to administer platelets prior to insertion to correct any deficits.
Respiratory function	Assessment of the patient's respiratory function may influence the choice of site, technique and type of device selected.
Septic profile	An elevated white blood cell count or raised temperature, possibly indicating an infection, could influence the type and timing of CVAD insertion. Antibiotic therapy may be required prior to insertion of a long-term access device.
Cardiovascular stability	This is desirable but not always possible and advice should be sought from the relevant physician, prior to insertion. In patients who require diuretics and restricted fluid intake, operational difficulties may arise as to location and cannulation of vessels, due to low central venous pressure.
Vascular status	Thrombosis, stenosis and anatomical anomalies may present difficulties for the operator.
Allergic status	This should be ascertained in order to eliminate any allergies to skin cleansing agents, sedatives, anaesthetics and dressings.

(Hamilton & Fermo 1998)

Financial considerations

An implanted port may not be approved for short-term therapies due to the higher costs associated with the insertion, although in the long term these devices may prove more cost effective than any other CVAD. There is also the cost associated with: personnel, use of a surgeon or anaesthetist; resources, such as theatre and radiology; anaesthetics; sedation; and X-rays. PICCs tend to incur lower costs as they are usually placed at the bedside by nurses (Winslow et al. 1995; Cole 1999; Hamilton 2000).

Decision-making tools can be useful to aid in the selection of the right CVAD for optimal clinical and financial benefits (Halderman 2000). Until recently there has been no systematic assessment tool or evidence-based guideline in the UK for VAD selection (Castledine 2002). There is now a decision-making model to enable proactive choice amongst healthcare professionals of the most appropriate VAD for patients, resulting in clinically effective intravenous therapy. This was developed by Bard and a group of nurses and is called AccessAbility (Bravery & Todd 2002; see Appendix 1). It took four years to complete, following an extensive literature review, and the model and educational programme includes:

- Anatomy and physiology of the venous system.
- Different types of VADs available and their advantages and disadvantages.
- Criteria for VAD selection.
- Algorithms to aid VAD selection.
- Interactive case histories to illustrate the process of VAD selection.
- Complications of intravenous therapy.
- History of VADs.
- Maintenance, care and complications of VADs.
- Drug information on pH and osmolarity.
- An audit tool containing VAD patient assessment forms, VAD outcomes and patient satisfaction questionnaire.

ANATOMY AND PHYSIOLOGY

The structure of the vein

The vein consists of three layers:

- Tunica intima is the innermost layer and in direct contact with venous flow. It is formed of a single layer of endothelial cells to provide a smooth surface that is non-thrombogenic. Damage to this layer can occur due to traumatic cannulation, irritation by stiff or large devices, as well as by irritant infusates and particulates. Any of these can result in platelet adherence and activation of the body's coagulation system. Within this layer are the valves, semi-lunar projections, which help to prevent the reflux of blood. Very large veins, such as the inferior and superior vena cava, do not have valves.
- Tunica media is the middle layer, which is composed of connective tissue containing muscular and elastic fibres. These enable veins to tolerate changes in pressure and flow by providing elastic recoil and muscular contraction.
- Tunica adventitia is the outer layer composed of longitudinal elastic fibres and loose connective tissue (Egan Sansivero 1998; Scales 1999; Hadaway 2001).

The main veins used for central venous access device placement vary in length and size (see Table 1.7).

The cephalic vein (see Fig. 1.1)
The cephalic vein ascends the outer border of the biceps muscle to the upper third of the arm and passes in the space between the pectoralis major and deltoid muscles. It terminates in the axillary vein, with a descending curve just below the clavicle, which can be connected to the external jugular or subclavian vein by a branch that passes upwards in front of the clavicle.

Table 1.7 Length and diameter of veins.

	Length (cm)	Diameter (mm)
Cephalic	38	6
Basilic	24	8
Axillary	13	16
Subclavian	6	19
Innominate	2.5	19
SVC	7	20

(Reproduced with permission from Egan Sansivero 1998)

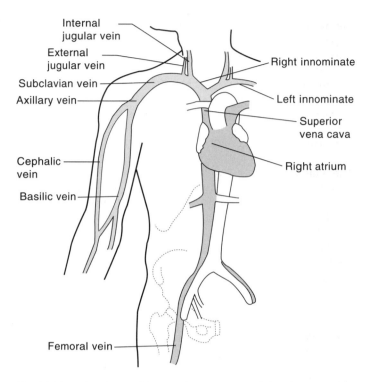

Fig. 1.1 The main veins used for central venous access device placement.

Advantages: it provides a straight and stable area for anchoring CVADs and is generally more comfortable.

Disadvantages: it is more tortuous than the basilic vein and presents greater potential for catheter tip malposition. The curvature is greater as it angles 90° to enter the terminal portion of the axillary vein, making advancement of a PICC difficult. (Egan Sansivero 1998; Hadaway 2001; Perucca 2001; Weinstein 2001).

The basilic vein (see Fig. 1.1)
The basilic vein is larger than the cephalic and originates in the ulnar aspect of the arm and tracts to the dorsal portion of the arm, where it is joined by the median cubital vein just above

the antecubital fossa. It ascends between the muscles in the upper arm to the axillary vein.

Advantages: it is usually the first choice for PICC insertion, as with arm at 90° it forms the straightest and most direct route into the central venous system. It is the largest vein in the upper arm and catheters up to 8 Fr (outer diameter) can be sited.

Disadvantages: more commonly malposition of the tip into the jugular vein (Egan Sansivero 1998; Hadaway 2001; Perucca 2001; Weinstein 2001).

The axillary vein (see Fig. 1.1)

This starts upwards as a continuation of the basilic vein, increasing in size as it ascends. It then receives the cephalic vein and terminates beneath the clavicle at the outer border of the first rib, becoming the subclavian vein (Egan Sansivero 1998; Hadaway 2001; Perucca 2001; Weinstein 2001). This vein can be used for the insertion of long-term catheters, but is not commonly used because identifying surface landmarks is difficult. However, infraclavicular axillary vein cannulation is possible using ultrasound guidance (Sharma et al. 2004).

The external jugular vein (see Fig. 1.1)

The posterior external jugular vein drains the occipital region and the anterior drains the ear – both join the external jugular vein at the base of the neck. The vein then follows the descending inward path to join the subclavian above the mid-clavicle region.

Advantages: it is observable and easily entered with a needle, making insertion complications rare.

Disadvantages: it varies in size and at its junction with the subclavian vein it is acutely angulated. The vein contains two pairs of valves, with the uppermost pair 4 cm above the clavicle, and the lower pair at the venous entrance to the subclavian vein. This can make advancement of the catheter more difficult.

A short catheter can be inserted easily using an introducer and a guidewire, and then directing the catheter to the ipsilateral nipple.

The contra-indications for using this route are (Egan Sansivero 1998; Hadaway 2001; Perucca 2001; Weinstein 2001):

- Catheter occlusion is a persistent problem, resulting from the patient's head movement.
- Venous phlebitis and possible dislodgement may also result from head movement, thereby reducing the life of the catheter.
- It can be hard to maintain an intact dressing to the area, due to movement, and beard growth on men.
- The idea of a catheter in the neck can be aesthetically and psychologically disturbing to many patients and their families.

The internal jugular vein (see Fig. 1.1)

This vein descends first behind and then to the outer side of the internal and common carotid arteries. The carotid plexus is situated on the outer side of internal carotid artery. The internal jugular joins the subclavian vein at the proximal root of the neck. At the angle of junction, the left subclavian receives the thoracic duct and the right receives the right lymphatic duct.

Advantages: the internal jugular vein is selected as the first choice due to its constant anatomical location, making it easier to catheterise than the subclavian. The right internal jugular vein is chosen as it forms a straighter, shorter line to the subclavian vein. Insertion is usually performed by first locating the vein with a small gauge needle, then making a small incision to facilitate the entry of a larger gauge catheter, which is inserted following the same direction as the introducer needle, aiming for the ipsilateral nipple.

Disadvantages: insertion could lead to damage of the carotid arteries and dressing of the catheter can be problematic (Egan Sansivero 1998; Hadaway 2001; Perucca 2001; Weinstein 2001).

The subclavian vein (see Fig. 1.1)

This vein is a continuation of the axillary vein and extends from the outer edge of the first rib to the inner end of clavicle, where it unites with the internal jugular vein to form the innominate vein. Valves are present in the venous system until about 2.5 cm before the innominate vein angles upwards and arches over the first rib, passing under the clavicle and forming a narrow passage for the vein. The apex of the lung is extremely close, thereby increasing the potential for pneumothorax when the subclavian is punctured, as well as increasing the chance of catheter compression between the clavicle and the first rib, known as 'pinch off' syndrome (Galloway & Bodenham 2004). *Advantages*: this route requires a short length of catheter, thus creating a high blood flow around a large portion of the catheter, which results in minimal irritation and obstruction. This, in turn, decreases the risk of complications and increases the life of the catheter. Entry may be performed by infra or supraclavicular approach. The catheter is inserted under the clavicle, aiming at the jugular notch (easily accessible for insertion and providing a flatter surface for dressing). The infraclavicular route is preferred in children, where the catheter is inserted about midpoint by the clavicle. The supraclavicular route is where the catheter is inserted at the base of a triangle formed by the sternal and clavicular heads of sternocleidomastoid muscle.

Disadvantages: both approaches are associated with pneumothorax, haemothorax and hydrothorax, brachial plexus injury and lymphatic duct injury.

Contra-indications include (Egan Sansivero 1998; Hadaway 2001; Perucca 2001; Weinstein 2001):

- radiation burns at intended insertion site;
- fractured clavicle;
- hyper-inflated lungs;
- malignant lesion at base of neck or apex of lungs;
- SVC syndrome;
- subclavian stenosis;
- history of central venous catheter placement problems.

The right and left innominate veins (also known as brachiocephalic veins) (see Fig. 1.1)

The right innominate is 2.5 cm long and carries blood vertically towards the thorax and joins the left innominate vein just below the cartilage of the first rib. The left innominate is 6 cm larger than the right and twice as long. It passes from left to right across the upper front chest in a downward slant and joins the right to form the SVC. The large lymphatic vessel receives a large quantity of lymph from the entire body and this may become damaged during puncture of large blood vessels in this area (Egan Sansivero 1998; Hadaway 2001; Perucca 2001; Weinstein 2001).

The superior vena cava (SVC) (see Fig. 1.1)

The SVC receives all the blood from the upper half of the body. It is composed of a short trunk 7 cm long and 2 cm wide. It begins below the first rib, close to the sternum on the right side, and then descends vertically, slightly to the right to the level of the third intercostal cartilage, where it empties into the right atrium of the heart. On chest X-ray its location is seen in the right mediastinal border. At the second costal space the fibrous pericardium of the heart begins and encompasses the lower half of the SVC. It also receives the azygous veins and small veins of the mediastinum, before passing into the right atrium. Other tributaries unite with the great thoracic veins and have been documented as an aberrant location for central venous catheters (Egan Sansivero 1998; Hadaway 2001; Perucca 2001; Weinstein 2001).

The right atrium (RA) (see Fig. 1.1)

The right atrium is one of two upper chambers of the heart and receives deoxygenated blood from the SVC, inferior vena cava (IVC) and the coronary sinus, where it then passes into the right ventricle (Anderson & Anderson 1995). Catheters which are advanced too far into the atrium can cause arrhythmias or an irregular heartbeat by stimulation of the arteroventricular or sinoatrial nodes (McPhee 1999; Macklin & Chernecky 2004).

The femoral vein (see Fig. 1.1)

The femoral vein is a continuation of the popliteal vein.
Advantages: femoral vein cannulation is the easiest to learn and perform, as the anatomy is predictable and the vein is large. It has its tip located in the inferior vena cava. There are few risks associated with its insertion (Seneff 1987a). This is an alternative site for emergencies and is a useful site for short-term catheterisation.

Disadvantages: it carries a high incidence of thrombus and increased infection rates once in situ (Egan Sansivero 1998; Hadaway 2001; Perucca 2001; Weinstein 2001).

GENERAL ASPECTS OF CVADs

Design of the device

Catheter material
The material selected is often dependent on the type of device and insertion procedure required. However, the composition and biocompatibility of the catheter material may influence development of central venous catheter-related complications, i.e. thrombus, vessel perforation and catheter-related blood-stream infections and therefore should be considered when making the device selection.

Type of material
Polyurethane and PVC were used in the past due to their stiff nature that allowed for easier percutaneous insertion. However, they are associated with increased thrombogenicity due to the rigidity of the catheter, which results in damage to the tunica intima and subsequent platelet aggregation and thrombus development. Polyurethane is now available as a rigid, semi-rigid and flexible material and is commonly used for short-term percutaneous central venous catheterisation. It can be stiff enough to allow for percutaneous insertion, but then softens after insertion, in response to the body temperature. This softening makes the catheter more biocompatible once in the vein. A variation is to compose the tip of another material, such as silicone, to reduce the possible damage to the lining of the vein on insertion. Polyurethane has tensile strength that permits the catheter to be constructed with thinner walls and smaller external diameters, thereby reducing the amount of foreign material within the vein. This also enables the catheter to tolerate higher infusion pressures, without having to sacrifice lumen size and the resultant decrease in flow capacity (Hadaway 1995).

Silastic is very soft biocompatible material that floats within the vein and is less likely to cause damage to the wall of the vessel. For this reason, the majority of long-term central venous catheters are constructed of silicone. The different mechanical properties of silicone necessitate thicker catheter walls to achieve strength; thus either the internal lumen size is decreased or the outer diameter is increased (Hadaway 1995).

All catheter material is radio opaque to allow for visualisation under fluoroscopy. Ease of visibility is related to the size of the catheter, radiological techniques and machine settings (Hadaway 1995). This is essential in order to determine the correct placement of the catheter and its tip after insertion, or whenever displacement/malposition is suspected.

Considerations

An important consideration when selecting the catheter material is that bacteria adhere to and multiply on the surface of catheters. Surface characteristics vary with different material. Many catheter surfaces appear smooth on visual inspection, but under an electron microscope surfaces are similar to lunar craters. Fibrin and bacteria adhere readily to these surfaces. A rough surface will result in an increased attachment of microorganisms and predispose to thrombus, which may further promote colonisation. Bacterial adherence varies with the type of catheter material (Elliott 1998).

Bacteria, such as coagulase negative staphylococcus, can excrete a polysaccharide material or 'slime' that coats the catheter and acts as an agent that bonds the organisms to the catheter. This slime layer or 'biofilm' renders systemic antibiotics ineffective (Ryder 2001). Another concern is the interaction of plasma proteins with the catheter surface. Within seconds of contact with the catheter surface, it is coated with body fluids and proteins, with subsequent platelet and fibrin disposition. Platelet disposition occurs on all foreign substances introduced into the vascular system and more takes place on some material than on others. Platelet adhesion and activation plays a major role toward thrombus formation. Catheters become encased by fibrin within 5–7 days, forming a fibrin sheath. Fibrin disposition occurs from the area where the catheter enters the skin to where its tip touches the intima of the vein (Vesely 2003).

In an effort to reduce these complications catheters have been coated or bonded with medications or antiseptics (Evans Orr 1993). Some may have an antibiotic bonded (e.g. minocycline/ rifampin) to the entire length of a catheter and the lumens, that provides protection against potential bacteria seeding on the catheter. Some are bonded with antiseptic material, such as silver sulfadiazine and chlorhexidine. All studies have been conducted using triple lumen non-cuffed catheters in adult patients whose catheters have remained in place less than 30 days. The benefits have been well established and they are recommended for use in high risk areas such as critical care units (DoH 2001; CDC 2002) (see Chapter 7). Improving catheter material by enhancing biocompatibility within the vein, e.g. hydromeric coated catheters as well as bonding catheters with heparin, may help to decrease thrombogenicity. The main disadvantage appears to be sensitivity.

Lumens
Devices are usually available with a number of lumens: single, double, triple and, in the case of non-tunnelled short-term catheters, even four and five lumens. This allows simultaneous infusion and administration of incompatible solutions and drugs. Consideration should be given to the flow rates achievable with each lumen and the configuration of the internal tip. An increase in the number of lumens is also associated with an increased risk of infection (DoH 2001).

Internal tip
There are two main types of tip endings in all catheters:

(1) *Open-ended*: an open-ended catheter can be of two designs. One type opens directly out at the end and can be cut to adjust the length of the catheter (see Fig. 1.2). The other has staggered openings to allow for a more flexible and less traumatic tip ending but cannot be cut (see Fig. 1.2). The main disadvantage of an open-ended catheter is the risk of blood reflux if it is not flushed effectively. In a multi-lumen catheter the openings are usually (Fig. 1.3):
(a) proximal, nearest patient;

(b) medial, middle;

(c) distal, furthest away from patient.

(2) *Valved*: there are two types of valved catheters, one with the valve in the tip, known as a Groshong valve (see Fig. 1.4) and the other has a valve in the hub, a PASV (pressure activated sensory valve) catheter (see Fig. 1.5). Valved catheters were developed to ensure that there is no blood reflux when the catheter is not in use. Both work on a pressure activated valve which opens with infusate (positive), and aspiration (negative), but remains closed in the absence of any pressure, and eliminates the need for clamping the device while connecting; therefore the catheters do not have clamps attached. For example, when drugs are administered either by injection or infusion the pressure created forces the valve open. When blood is withdrawn the valve opens to allow blood withdrawal. The pressure needed to cause the valve to open is high during the aspiration process and higher than typically present in the venous system, thereby reducing the incidence of blood reflux during disconnects and/or if the infusion bag runs dry.

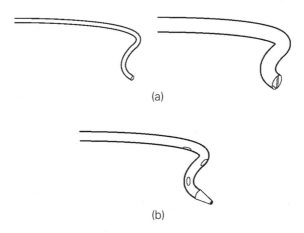

(a)

(b)

Fig. 1.2 Types of catheter tip. (a) Open ended catheter (single and double lumen), (b) staggered exit open ended catheter.

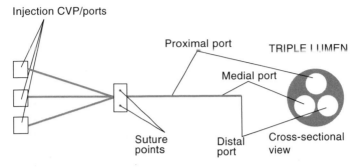

Fig. 1.3 Cross-sectional view of open ended triple lumen CVC. Reproduced with permission of the RCN from Quick Reference Guide 6, *Nursing Standard*, **13** (42).

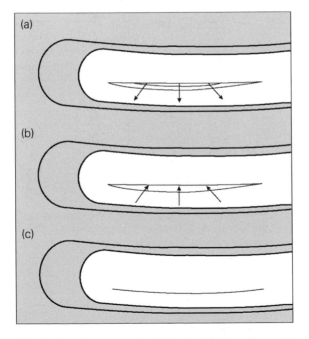

Fig. 1.4 The Groshong® two-way valve. (a) Infusion (positive pressure), (b) aspiration (negative pressure), (c) closed (neutral pressure).

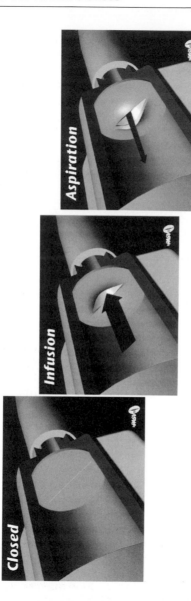

Fig. 1.5 Pressure activated sensory valve (PASV) catheter. Brown Scientific.

Hoffman (1998) provided an overview of the valves' effective-ness, and this was further supported by Inwood (1999), who in a small study showed the impact the device could have at reducing occlusion. Hoffer et al. (1999) studied the incidence of occlusion, infection and malfunction when comparing valved with non-valved PICCs. They found a statistically significant difference in the complication rate for the valved PICCs, showing that occlusion and infection were reduced and the catheters did not require a heparin flush. However, there still appears to be a problem with clot formation and persistent withdrawal occlu-sion. Mayo et al. (1996) found that the addition of a heparinised saline flush decreased the presence of intraluminal adherence clots and improved catheter function. In some cases, when com-paring valved and open-ended catheters no difference has been noted in both the early or late complications in ports (Biffi et al. 2001) or catheters (Tolar & Gould 1996).

Length of catheter
Catheters are manufactured in a variety of lengths and many can be trimmed to suit the needs of the patient either at the internal tip or the distal end. Total length of the catheter may include the length advanced into the vein, the hub and connector and any portion not intended for insertion into the vein. This information is important when determining accurate measurements of inter-nal volume and indicating any dislodgement of the device.

Diameter
The catheter size is usually measured in French or gauge. French size equals the outside diameter of the catheter in mm multi-plied by three. Gauge measurements may be used to measure the outer or inner diameter and range from 13–28 gauge, with the smallest number indicating the largest size (Hadaway 1995). The outer diameter is important in relation to the diameter of the vein lumen. If the catheter is too large for the vessel, blood flow around the catheter may be inadequate for the dilution of any infusate or medication, and motion against the vein wall can both result in chemical and mechanical irritation. Internal diameters are important to ascertain the internal volume, flow capabilities and pressure ratings (Hadaway 1995).

Cuffs

Cuffs made of Dacron® are usually found on tunnelled catheters. They remain in the subcutaneous tissue several centimetres away from the insertion site on the skin. They provide a mechanical barrier to the migration of micro-organisms and as the tissue grows into the cuff this aids in the fixation of the device (Hadaway 1995). There are now cuffs, which contain silver ions, to provide anti-microbial activity, although studies have not shown any great benefits (CDC 2002).

GENERAL ASPECTS RELATED TO INSERTION

Who should insert CVADs?

Insertion of central venous access devices may be undertaken by either a nurse, or a doctor, who has received adequate training and supervision. In the past the act of inserting a central venous catheter was always performed by doctors, usually anaesthetists, surgeons or radiologists. However, in the last ten years this area of expert practice has been developed by nurses in the UK. PICC insertion by nurses first began in the USA in the late 1980s and was developed in some oncology units in the UK in the early 1990s. At the same time a few nurse specialists trained in the insertion of skin-tunnelled catheters and developed nurse-led services for CVAD insertions. The advantages are summarised below, illustrated using the evidence generated by the nurses in practice.

Nurse-led services

Hamilton et al. (1995) found that the timing of CVAD placements was unreliable and this, in turn, delayed the nutritional support required by patients or those who were immunosuppressed. Patients also became frustrated due to cancellation and felt that there was lack of continuity of care by ward nurses. They found that there were problems related to infection rates and increased complication rates associated with insertion by inexperienced practitioners. There was an issue with costs, which included theatre costs, increased length of stay due to complications, and correction of misplacement, as well as the use of unfamiliar and expensive products. They introduced a nurse-led service for the insertion of skin-tunnelled catheters and once the service was established they were able to demonstrate a low complication rate, with only 1% of patients suffering from a pneumothorax and a 1% sepsis rate over the period of one year. The service has now expanded and is able to support a full training programme for other nurses and doctors (Hamilton 2004).

Fitzsimmons et al. (1997) trained a clinical nurse specialist to insert tunnelled CVCs according to predetermined guidelines. The CVCs were inserted in the outpatient department under local anaesthetic and compared with services provided by junior medical staff. The main outcome measures were the success of the procedure; and reduction in insertion-related infection rates and waiting times. Rates of failed insertions fell from 20% to 3% (and there was a reduction in surgical referrals). The waiting time for 97% of patients was reduced to less than one working day compared with 80% previously. Infection rates in the first 30 days after insertion fell from 10 per 72 to 2 per 200. They concluded that the nurse specialist had improved the quality of service and gave junior doctors more support and opportunities to become competent.

Benton & Marsden (2002) examined the training of nurses placing tunnelled catheters using imaging techniques of real time sonography and fluoroscopy and its implication for practice. Previously CVCs for haematology patients were inserted under general anaesthetic by doctors. When practice was reviewed it was found that of the 13 doctors who placed CVCs (n = 96) there was a rate of 6% procedure-related complications when using the subclavian route. They found that by training nurses and using sonography to guide vessel puncture it improved the success rate of insertion and reduced the complication rate.

Kelly (2003) developed a team who inserted all catheters within an X-ray department using ultrasound guidance and found that it improved the service, reduced waiting times and patients appeared to be pleased with the care. Boland et al. (2003) examined the clinical and cost effectiveness of blind insertion by nurses. They randomised 470 adult cancer patients to receive blind or image-guided skin-tunnelled catheter insertion. Blind insertion was without the use of image guidance at any point in the procedure and took place at the patient's bedside. Image-guided placement was performed in the interventional X-ray suite and the position of the guidewire was checked before the catheter was inserted, which was then positioned with use of X-ray fluoroscopy. Both interventions involved blind venepuncture of the subclavian vein. There was no statistically significant difference between the mean cost. The only statistically significant difference in clinical outcomes was the frequency of catheter tip misplacement. It was higher in the blind arm, where 14% had misplaced tips, when compared with 1% under image guidance. It was also evident that nurses previously inexperienced in the procedure could be trained within a three-month period, to insert tunnelled catheters successfully both at the bedside and under guidance. Patient satisfaction was also high.

Where should insertion be performed?

The location has often been dictated by the practitioner, surgeons and anaesthetists tend to perform insertions in a theatre setting or in critical care/A & E units. Radiologists usually insert devices under X-ray guidance in an interventional suite within the radiology department. Nurses have not always had access to these areas and so began placing at the bedside, with no increase in infection rates (Hamilton et al. 1995). This frees up other areas required for alternative aspects of care and is also less anxiety provoking for the patient.

How should insertion be performed?

There are some basic steps to inserting a central venous access device, which are common to all insertions:

(1) preparation of the practitioner;
(2) sterile procedure;
(3) skin cleansing;
(4) position of the patient;
(5) use of ultrasound;
(6) use of anaesthetic;
(7) tip placement;
(8) radiological confirmation;
(9) documentation.

Preparation of the practitioner
Handwashing is a key element in the preparation process. CVADs are associated with a high risk of infection so the first step is good handwashing and the use of sterile gloves.

Sterile procedure
There is no doubt that the insertion of a CVAD should be performed using a strict aseptic technique, that is the practitioners wearing a sterile gown, sterile gloves, in some cases a mask and goggles (these are often used more for protection of the practitioner than providing protection for the patients from the risk of infection), and the use of large sterile drapes (Elliott 1993; Elliott et al. 1994).

Skin cleansing
There are many cleaning solutions available and there is much confusion as to the best solution. Maki et al. (1991) carried out a study comparing three cleaning solutions for use prior to the insertion of CVC and arterial catheters. These were chlorhexidine 2% aqueous solution, 70% isopropyl alcohol and povidone iodine. They found that the best cleaning solution was chlorhexidine. This is because it provides the most effective disinfection of micro-organisms and combines the benefits of rapid action with excellent residual activity (Pellowe et al. 2004). The 2% solution has been difficult to obtain in the UK, and most hospitals use 0.5% chlorhexidine in alcohol. Alcohol is also an effective cleaning solution and it dries quickly. The key to effective site disinfection is using the correct cleaning solution; applying it in the right way for the correct amount of time; and allowing it to air-dry completely. Elliott et al. (1994) stated that drying should be for up to 30 seconds, but may take longer. Drying is vital if disinfection is to be achieved. Inserting a device through wet skin results in a stinging sensation for the patient and an inadequately prepared skin surface. This enables bacteria to travel through the skin directly into the venous system, thereby increasing the chance of infection.

Shaving: The issue of whether to shave prior to inserting a CVAD is a thorny one. It is believed that adequate skin cleansing results

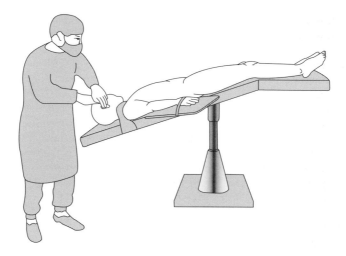

Fig. 1.6 The Trendelenberg position. Redrawn with permission from Drewett, S. (2000) Central venous catheter removal. *British Journal of Nursing*, **9** (22), 2308.

in adequate cleansing of the hair over the area. Shaving usually results in skin abrasions, which could become contaminated and cause infections. If skin is to be shaved it should be done with an electric razor or the hair should be clipped with a pair of scissors (McPhee 1999; INS 2000; RCN 2003).

Position of the patient (see Fig. 1.6)
Patients should be positioned to enable easy access to the site and to optimise venous filling. This may be achieved by tilting the patient head down to enable filling of the jugular vessels, known as the Trendelenberg position (see Chapter 3). The patient's head may also need to be turned toward to site of PICC insertion to prevent jugular placement.

Use of ultrasound
The use of two-dimensional ultrasound imaging is now recommended by NICE (2002) for all routine placements of central venous access devices. The National Institute for Clinical Excellence (NICE) carried out a health technology appraisal on

ultrasound locating devices for the placing of central venous catheters. Venous access has traditionally been achieved by puncturing a central vein and passing the needle along the anticipated line of the relevant vein, by using surface anatomical landmarks. This is known as the 'landmark method'. Whilst experienced operators using the landmark method can achieve relatively high success rates with few complications, failure rates as high as 35% have been reported in the literature (NICE 2002). The most common complications include pneumothorax, arterial puncture, nerve injury and multiple unsuccessful attempts.

Ultrasound technology has been used in interventional radiology to guide other percutaneous procedures. It provides the operator with visualisation of the desired vein and surrounding structures before and during insertion, as well as detection of anatomical variants and thrombosis within the vessel. It also has the potential to reduce complications. Fig. 1.7 shows an ultrasound machine.

Two types of real time ultrasound imaging guidance are available:

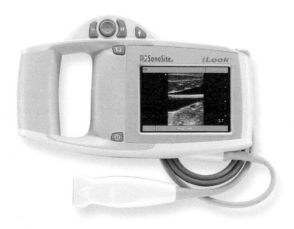

Fig. 1.7 Two-dimensional imaging ultrasound machine. Image courtesy of Sonosite Ltd.

- two-dimensional imaging ultrasound guidance;
- audio-guided Doppler ultrasound guidance.

Two dimensional ultrasound is favoured. Portable ultrasound machines are now available and can be used anywhere in the hospital setting. However, operators need to be trained in the use of this equipment. Following an extensive literature review the report made the following recommendations:

- two-dimensional imaging ultrasound guidance is recommended as the preferred method of insertion of CVADs into the internal jugular vein in adults and children in elective situations (Calvert et al. 2003; Mey et al. 2003).
- The use of two-dimensional imaging ultrasound guidance should be considered in most clinical circumstances where CVAD insertion is necessary, whether electively or in an emergency situation.
- It is recommended that all those involved in placing CVADs using two-dimensional imaging ultrasound guidance should undertake appropriate training to achieve competence.
- Audio-guided Doppler ultrasound is not recommended for CVAD insertion.

All NHS trusts in which CVADs are used, all those who routinely insert CVADs and those responsible for clinical training programmes had to review policies and procedures and identify the number of two-dimensional imaging ultrasound units required and appropriate locations for each unit. They also had to train a sufficient number of healthcare professionals from a range of disciplines in the proper use of the units and identify the financial and service implications of implementing the guidance. Finally, trusts had to recognise that the decision to use two-dimensional imaging ultrasound guidance or landmark method continues to be informed by:

- Competence and previous experience of the operator.
- Anatomical site of the CVC insertion and other anticipated technical difficulties.
- Urgency of clinical need.

Use of anaesthetic

There are a number of methods of reducing pain and anxiety during CVAD placement. These include injectable or topical local anaesthetics, sedation, general anaesthetic, as well as use of relaxation techniques, distraction and anxiolytics (Moureau & Zonderman 2000).

Local anaesthetic

Topical: The use of local anaesthetic has been advocated to reduce pain and anxiety (Dougherty & Lamb 1999; Moureau & Zonderman 2000) and can be applied in a cream/gel, or given as an intradermal injection. The most commonly used local anaesthetic creams are EMLA™ (Eutectic Mixture of Local Anaesthetics: Lidocaine and prilocaine) and Ametop™ (topical amethocaine). These are applied to the skin 30–60 minutes prior to venepuncture and covered with an occlusive dressing. EMLA™ can cause vasoconstriction, making venepuncture more difficult. Ametop™ has been shown to be more effective than EMLA™ and causes significantly less vasoconstriction (Brown 1999). However, application can result in an erythmatous rash if left in situ longer than the recommended time (BMA/RPS 2005).

Injectable Lidocaine: Lidocaine (lignocaine) is a widely used local anaesthetic agent and its main site of action is the nerve membrane. The onset of Lidocaine is rapid and duration of action is intermediate (Boyle 2003). Intradermal Lidocaine 1% can be slowly injected around the vein prior to insertion or subcutaneously around the area prepared for tunnelling. However, it should be used with caution due to its potential for allergic reaction, tissue damage and inadvertent injection of drug into the vascular system. It can also obliterate the vein when administered prior to PICC insertion (INS 2000; Perucca 2001). It is routinely used during micropuncture insertion of PICCs and for non-tunnelled and tunnelled CVAD insertion.

Sedation: Conscious sedation is often used when tunnelled catheters are inserted. The sedation is usually administered intravenously and the commonest drug is midazolam. This is a non-irritant drug and is produced as 10 mg in 5 ml, which allows for easier titration (i.e. giving the drug slowly in very small amounts while watching the patient's response (Boyle 2003).

The main effects are on the:

- Central nervous system: midazolam can cause depression, which is dose related, the clinical effect varying between different drugs. It can also cause hypnosis, amnesia, is a muscle relaxant and anticonvulsant. The amnesia produced is anterograde, which means patients will not remember events occurring after the injection, although they will recall what happens before the drug takes effect. Lack of memory is a definite advantage and lasts 20–30 minutes, but can vary, so patients and carers should be warned that care will be required up to eight hours (Boyle 2003; Craig 2003).
- Respiratory system may become depressed, although this is usually mild and insignificant in normal healthy patients and when the drug is administered intravenously by slow titration, but can be significant in patients who are unwell, have impaired respiratory function, are on CNS depressants, such as opioids, and the elderly. It is therefore important to monitor respirations during sedation, both clinically (depth and rate of breathing), and using a pulse oximeter to provide a non-invasive method of continuous monitoring of the patient's pulse and oxygen saturation (Boyle 2003; Craig 2003).
- Cardiovascular system: the effects are slight and insignificant in healthy patients, but may present as a fall in blood pressure and increase in heart rate immediately after injection. Even in cardiovascularly compromised individuals, these are not usually a problem when a slow titration method is used to produce sedation (Boyle 2003).

The main advantages of using midazolam are:

- rapid onset (3–4 minutes);
- adequate patient cooperation;
- good amnesic.

The main disadvantages are:

- not an analgesic;
- causes respiratory depression;

- disinhibition effects occasionally occur;
- post-operative supervision required for eight hours, due to sedation and muscle relaxant effects;
- not suitable for sedating children;
- the elderly are easily over sedated.

Contra-indications include (Craig 2003):

- pregnancy/breast feeding;
- severe psychosis;
- alcohol/drug abuse;
- impairment of hepatic function;
- the patient is unable to provide an escort if going home following sedation.

Administration and monitoring: When administering sedation the patient should be warned of a cold sensation at the cannula site. A suitable administration regimen is 2 mg (1 ml) injected over 30 seconds, followed by a pause of 90 seconds and then further increments of 1 mg (0.5 mls) every 30 seconds until sedation is judged to be adequate. Throughout this time the nurse must talk to the patient and observe for any adverse reactions. The correct dose has been given when there is slurring of speech and slowed response to commands. Patients over 65 require lower doses.

Monitoring should include depth and rate of respirations, remembering that oxygen saturation is 97–100% (lower in smokers, the elderly and those with respiratory disease). Oxygen should be administered to all sedated patients (BSGE 2003). It is important to ensure that reversal agents are available. Flumazenil (Arexate) can reverse the sedation, cardiovascular and respiratory depression, but not the amnesic. It is usually recommended for use only in emergency situations (Craig 2003).

Sedation is not always necessary. Kelly (2003) did not routinely sedate her patients undergoing tunnelled catheter insertion. Instead she used injectable local anaesthetic and talked to her patients during the procedure, providing comfort and support. Patients were told that they could be sedated if they requested it. Most ports are placed under a general anaesthetic.

Tip placement

The direction and degree of tip movement is dependent on several variables including:

- the type of catheter;
- insertion site;
- size of patient.

The final position of a PICC is dependent on the insertion site and the position of the patient's arm; and the catheter can move at least 2 cm further into the right atrium on movement (Forauer & Alonzo 2000). If placed in the left arm it can move more than in the right and when placed in the basilic vein it moves more than if in the cephalic vein (Vesely 2003). Anatomical changes occur with subclavian and internal jugular insertion when the patient sits upright following insertion and the catheter tip can move upward. In a skin-tunnelled catheter this can be 2–3 cm, especially in female patients with substantial breast tissue, and overweight patients of either sex. Large diameter catheters can move more than smaller ones and subclavian more than internal jugular placements. A correctly placed catheter tip will be likely to be one that undergoes a range of movement between the SVC and upper RA.

The tip location will affect the catheter performance: if the tip is too high it may be sucked against the adjacent wall when aspiration is applied, or if the tip is too far within the RA (Vesely 2002, 2003). A catheter tip positioned against a vascular wall may also become a source of persistent irritation, leading to denudation of the vascular endothelium and creation of a potential nidus for thrombus formation (Mayo 2001; Galloway & Bodenham 2004). This is reported more frequently in patients who have left-sided placements (Perdue 2001). The arguments for right atrial tip placements are that the tip is in a large chamber preventing contact, and blood flow prevents accumulation of thrombin and minimises irritation of substances. The disadvantages of this tip position are an increase in cardiac arrhythmias (although this may be associated with the insertion of the guidewire as it is reduced when insertion is performed using imaging combined with cardiac monitoring), and catheter induced perforation, which is also reduced by using softer materials and imaging guidance (Vesely 2002). A study of non-tunnelled CVCs compared the standard method (15 cm from insertion site) with a tailored method of measuring distance to determine depth. This new method significantly reduced the frequency of CVC tips entering the right atrium. The distance between the distal and proximal ports of multilumen CVCs was also taken into consideration in order to decrease the risk of extravasation via the proximal port (Chalkiadis & Goucke 1998).

Radiological confirmation of tip placement

A chest X-ray must always be performed following CVAD placement, to verify tip location and to ensure that there is no pneumothorax. This must be documented so that any practitioner using the device will know that the X-ray has been seen and checked and that the device is safe to use. This is recommended by both the INS (2000) and the RCN (2003). However, there is some debate over the relevance in some cases.

The landmarks used for chest radiography assist in determining tip location (Wise et al. 2001) (see Fig. 1.8):

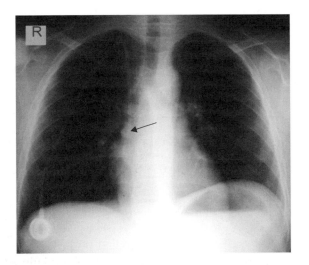

Fig. 1.8 Chest X-ray illustrating tip location of catheter in lower SVC (arrow).

- airway passages: trachea, bronchi, trachiobronchial angle and carina;
- bony structures: clavicle, ribs, scapula, sternum;
- cardiac silhouette: SVC, pulmonary vessels, aortic arch, and azygous arch;
- artriocaval junction, IVC and RV;
- diaphragm.

Most chest X-rays are performed using the posterior anterior (PA) view. Royer (2001) suggested that there was a need for taking both the PA and lateral view. The lateral view can confirm or rule out an aberrant tip location missed on frontal projection, by detecting malposition that may not be identified on PA position (Wise et al. 2001).

Documentation

There are a number of aspects that should be documented following the insertion of any CVAD. This enables continuity of care but also the ability to manage and problem solve any issues related to the device. First, information regarding the type of device, the manufacturer, the size and the lot number and expiry date should be recorded. This is vital in order to be able to track devices, particularly if there is a fault found with the device itself or a device recall. Both the original and trimmed (where appropriate) length of the catheter, as well as actual length inserted and external length at insertion site will all aid in determining correct position and identifying if there has been any movement which may alert the practitioner to a tip malposition.

Second, the specific vein used and insertion technique, such as the use of ultrasound, should be documented, along with any problems during insertion that occurred using any other veins. This is invaluable if another practitioner needs to replace a device as they can then avoid using veins where there have been previous problems. Other aspects that should be documented are if a sedative or local anaesthetic is used, and if so the type, volume or dose required, with a section on how the patient tolerated the procedure; the flush solution used and the amount; the appearance of the catheter site, for example if there is any bruising; the type of securement device and dressing applied and if this is different from standard practice give the reason why, e.g. patient allergic to transparent dressings; and dressing applied.

Finally, if the patient has been sent for an X-ray, document that the X-ray has been seen and verify the tip location. If the patient is to be discharged with the device in situ then any teaching given to the patient and/or carer, the type of written information and equipment given and where appropriate if the district nurses have been informed, should all be documented in the nursing notes (Weinstein 2001).

ISSUES RELATED TO PATIENT CONSENT

Patients have the right to be informed about all available options, significant risks and treatment options (McDermott 1995). Consent for any invasive procedure is vital, but for a device that is associated with hazards on insertion and complications once in situ, it is imperative that the patient fully understands all aspects of the procedure. Ideally, a patient should be assessed and all types of devices discussed, covering all the advantages and disadvantages of each type, and a full explanation should be given of the procedure involved for insertion. This should be supported by written information that the patient can take home and read, with their family where appropriate, and then make a final informed decision. Contact numbers should also be given to the patient to enable them to phone and discuss any issues prior to making the decision or attending for the procedure.

Where the patient will not have a choice, e.g. when having a CVAD for surgery, then the device should be shown to the patient and an explanation given as to its management once in situ.

Just prior to the procedure, time should be taken to repeat all the information and reinforce the risks. The patient should then be given time to ask any questions and to read in full the consent form. See Appendix 2 for an example of a pre-printed consent form for PICC insertion. The patient is then required to sign the form and a copy should be made so that one copy is filed in the patient's notes and the other is given to the patient to keep for reference.

Scenario

A 30-year-old man with Crohn's disease is admitted to start parenteral nutrition and has been told he will require a long-term central venous access device. He is married with two young children and up until his illness progressed, he enjoyed playing tennis and taking his children swimming.

What CVADs would you think would be most suitable for him and what aspects of each will you discuss with him?

The three main devices of choice are a PICC, a skin-tunnelled catheter and a port. There are advantages and disadvantages to each. The port would be suitable as he likes to swim, but this would require him accessing the port each day to set up his PN infusion. A PICC may restrict his tennis playing, he would not be able to swim and it may get pulled when he plays with the children. A tunnelled catheter would restrict his swimming but may be the best option for delivery of his therapy. Once he has had all the pros and cons explained he could then make an informed choice as to which device to select.

CONCLUSION

There are a large variety of central venous access devices that can be selected, but it is important to assess the patient prior to insertion to ensure that the most suitable device is used. This increases compliance by the patient with all aspects of the care and management of the device, as well as providing the means for therapy whilst enhancing their quality of life.

REFERENCES

Anderson, K.N. & Anderson, L.E. (1995) *Mosby Pocket Dictionary of Nursing, Medicine and Professions Allied to Medicine*, UK edn. Mosby, London.

Benton, S. & Marsden, C. (2002) Training nurses to place tunnelled central venous catheters. *Professional Nurse*, **17** (9), 531–535.

Biffi, R., De Brand, F., Orsi, F., Pozzi, S., Arnaldi, P., Goldhirsch, A., Rotmensz, N., Robertson, C., Bellomi, M. & Andreoni, M. (2001)

A randomised prospective trial of central venous ports connected to standard open-ended or Groshong catheters in adult oncology patients. *Cancer*, **92** (5), 1204–1212.

Boland, A., Haycox, A., Bagust, A. & Fitzsimmons, L. (2003) A randomised controlled trial to evaluate the clinical and cost effectiveness of Hickman line insertion in adult cancer patients by nurses. *Health Technology Assessment*, **7**, 36.

Boyle, C. (2003) Chapter 2 Physiology and pharmacology of sedation agents. In: Skelly, M. & Palmer, D. (eds) *Conscious Sedation in Gastroenterology: a Handbook for Nurse Practitioners.* pp. 17–34. Whurr Publishers, London.

Bravery, K. & Todd, J. The AccessAbility™ programme website (2002). Bard Limited London: www.accessibiltybybard.co.uk

British Medical Association and Royal Pharmaceutical Society (2005) *British National Formulary*. British Medical Association and Royal Pharmacological Society, London.

British Society of Gastroenterology (BSGE) (2003) *Safety and Sedation During Endoscopic Procedures*. BSGE, London.

Brown, J. (1999) Topical Ametocaine (Ametop™) is superior to EMLA™ for intravenous cannulation. *Canadian Journal of Anaesthetics*, **46**, 1014–1018.

Calvert, N., Hind, D., McWilliams, R.G., Thomas, S.M., Beverly, C. & Davidson, A. (2003) The effectiveness and cost effectiveness of ultrasound locating devices for central venous access: a systematic review and economic evaluation. *Health Technology Assessment*, **7** (12).

Carlson, K.R. (1999) Correct utilisation and management of PICCs and midline catheters in the alternate care setting. *Journal of Intravenous Nursing*, **22** (supplement 6), S46–S50.

Castledine, G. (2002) New initiative to provide evidence based intravenous care. *British Journal of Nursing*, **11** (20), 1351.

Center for Disease Control and Prevention (2002) Guidelines for the prevention of intravascular catheter related infections. *Morbidity and Mortality Weekly Report*, **51** (RR10), 1–26.

Chalkiadis, G.A. & Goucke, C.R. (1998) Depth of central venous catheter insertion in adults: an audit and assessment of a technique to improve tip position. *Anaesthetic and Intensive Care*, (26), 61–66.

Chernecky, C., Macklin, D., Nugent, K. & Waller, J.L. (2002) The need for shared decision making in the selection of vascular access devices: an assessment of patients and clinicians. *Journal of Vascular Access Devices*, **7** (3), 34–39.

Clinical Haematology Task Force (1997) Guidelines on the insertion and management of central venous lines. *British Journal of Haematology*, (98), 1041–1047.

Cole, D. (1999) Selection and management of central venous access devices in the home setting. *Journal of Intravenous Nursing*, **22** (6), 315–319.

Craig, D. (2003) Chapter 4 Clinical Techniques. In: Skelly, M. & Palmer, D. (eds) *Conscious Sedation in Gastroenterology: a Handbook for Nurse Practitioners*, pp. 50–67. Whurr Publishers, London.

Davidson, T. & Al-Mufti, R. (1997) Hickman central venous catheters in cancer patients. *Cancer Topics*, **10** (8), 10–14.

Department of Health (2001) Guidelines for preventing infections associated with the insertion and maintenance of central venous catheters. *Journal of Hospital Infection*, **47** (supplement), S47–S67.

Dougherty, L. & Lamb, J. (1999), *Intravenous Therapy in Nursing Practice*. Churchill Livingstone, Edinburgh.

Dougherty, L. & Lister, S. (2004) *The Royal Marsden Manual of Clinical Nursing Procedures*, 6th edn. Blackwell Science, Oxford.

Egan Sansivero, G. (1998) Venous anatomy and physiology. Considerations for vascular access device placement and function. *Journal of Intravenous Nursing*, **21** (supplement 5), S107–S114.

Elliott, T.S.J. (1993) Line associated bacteraemias. *Public Health Laboratories Service Communicable Disease Report*, **3** (7), R91–R96.

Elliott, T.S.J. (1998) Prevention of central venous catheter related infection. *Journal of Hospital Infection*, **40**, 193–201.

Elliott, T.S.J., Faroqui, M.H., Armstrong, R.F. & Hanson, G.C. (1994) Guidelines for good practice in central venous catheterisation. *Journal of Hospital Infection*, **28**, 163–176.

Evans Orr, M. (1993) Issues in management of peripheral central venous catheters. *Nursing Clinics of North America*, **28** (4), 911–918.

Fitzsimmons, C.L., Gilleece, M.H., Ranson, M.R., Wardley, A., Morris, C. & Scarffe, J.H. (1997). Central venous catheter placement: extending the role of the nurse. *Journal of the Royal College of Physicians*, **31** (5), 533–535.

Forauer, A.R. & Alonzo, M. (2000) Change in peripherally inserted central catheter tip position with abduction and adduction of the upper extremity. *Journal of Vascular and Interventional Radiology*, **11**, 1315–1318.

Galloway, S. & Bodenham, A. (2004) Long-term central venous access. *British Journal of Anaesthesia*, **92**, 722–734.

Goodwin, M. & Carlson, I. (1993) The peripherally inserted central catheter: a retrospective look at three years of insertions. *Journal of Intravenous Nursing*, **16** (2), 92–103.

Hadaway, L.C. (1995) Comparison of vascular access devices. *Seminars in Oncology Nursing*, **11** (3), 154–166.

Hadaway, L.C. (2001) Anatomy and physiology. In: Carlson, K., Perdue, M.B. & Hankins, J. (eds) *Infusion Therapy in Clinical Practice*, 2nd edn. W.B. Saunders, Pennsylvania.

Halderman, F. (2000) VAD: selecting a vascular access device. *Nursing*, **30** (11), 59–61.

Hamilton, H. (2000) Selecting the correct intravenous device: nursing assessment. *British Journal of Nursing*, **9** (15), 960–970.

Hamilton, H. (2004) Advantages of a nurse-led central venous vascular access service. *Journal of Vascular Access*, **5**, 109–112.

Hamilton, H. & Fermo, K. (1998) Assessment of patients requiring intravenous therapy via a central venous route. *British Journal of Nursing*, **7** (8), 451–460.

Hamilton, H., O'Byrne, M. & Nicholai, L. (1995) Central lines inserted by clinical nurse specialists. *Nursing Times*, **91** (17), 38–39.

Hoffer, E.K., Borsa, J., Santulli, P., Bloch, R. & Fontaine, A.B. (1999) Prospective randomised comparison of valved versus non-valved peripherally inserted central venous catheters. *American Journal of Radiology*, (173), 1393–1398.

Hoffman, S. (1998) Valved catheters. *Journal of Vascular Access Devices*, (Summer), 18–19.

Intravenous Nursing Society (INS) (2000) *Standards for Infusion Therapy.* Beckon Dickinson and Intravenous Nursing Society, Massachusetts, USA.

Inwood, S. (1999) A preliminary assessment of an innovative valved catheter. *Journal of Vascular Access Devices*, (Summer), 30–32.

Jackson, A. (2003) Reflecting on the nursing contribution to vascular access. *British Journal of Nursing*, **12** (11), 657–665.

Kelly, L.J. (2003) A nurse-led service for tunnelled central venous catheter insertion. *Nursing Times*, **99** (38), 26–29.

McDermott, M.K. (1995) Patient education and compliance issues associated with access devices. *Seminars in Oncology Nursing*, **11** (3), 221–226.

Macklin, D. & Chernecky, C. (2004), *Intravenous Therapy.* Saunders, St Louis.

Maki, D.G., Ringer, M. & Alvarado, C.J. (1991) Prospective randomised trial of povidone-iodine alcohol and chlorhexidine for prevention of infection associated with central venous and arterial catheters. *The Lancet*, **338**, 339–343.

Mayo, D.J. (2001) Catheter related thrombosis. *Journal of Intravenous Nursing*, **24** (supplement 3), S13–S20.

Mayo, D.J., Horne, M.K., Summers, B.L., Pearson, D.C. & Helsabeck, C.B. (1996) The effects of heparin flush on patency of the Groshong catheter: a pilot study. *Oncology Nursing Forum*, **23** (9), 1401–1405.

McPhee, A. (1999) *Handbook of Infusion Therapy.* Springhouse Corporation, Pennsylvania.

Mey, U., Glasmacher, A., Hahn, C., Gorschulter, M., Ziske, C., Mergelsberg, M., Sauerbruch, T. & Schmidt-Wolf, I.G.H. (2003)

Evaluation of an ultrasound-guided technique for central venous access via the internal jugular vein in 493 patients. *Supportive Care in Cancer*, (11), 148–155.

Moureau, N. & Zonderman, A. (2000) Does it always have to hurt? *Journal of Intravenous Nursing*, **23** (4), 213–219.

National Association of Vascular Access Network (1998) Tip location of peripherally inserted central catheters. *Journal of Vascular Access Devices*, **3** (2), 8–10.

National Institute for Clinical Excellence (2002) *Ultrasound Locating Devices for Placing a Central Venous Line* (Oct.). National Institute for Clinical Excellence, London.

Perdue, M.B. (2001) Intravenous complications. In: Carlson, K., Perdue, M.B. & Hankins, J. (eds) *Infusion Therapy in Clinical Practice*, 2nd edn. W.B. Saunders, Pennsylvania.

Pellowe, C.M., Pratt, R.J., Loveday, H.P., Harper, P., Robinson, N. & Jones, S.R.L. (2004) The *epic* project. Updating the evidence base for national evidence-based guidelines for preventing healthcare–associated infection in NHS hospitals in England: a report with recommendations. *British Journal of Infection Control* **5** (6), 10–16.

Perucca, R. (2001) Obtaining vascular access. In: Carlson, K., Perdue, M.B. & Hankins, J. (eds) *Infusion Therapy in Clinical Practice*, 2nd edn. W.B. Saunders, Pennsylvania.

Royal College of Nursing Intravenous Therapy Forum (2003) *RCN Standards for Infusion Therapy*. Royal College of Nursing, London.

Royer, T. (2001) A case for posterior, anterior, and lateral chest X-rays being performed following each PICC placement. *Journal of Vascular Access Devices*, **6** (4), 9–11.

Ryder, M. (2001) The role of biofilm in vascular catheter related infections. *New Developments in Vascular Diseases*, **2** (2), 15–21.

Scales, K. (1999) Vascular access in the acute care setting. In: Dougherty, L. & Lamb J. (eds) *Intravenous Therapy in Nursing Practice*. Churchill Livingstone, Edinburgh.

Seneff, M.G. (1987a) Central venous catheterisation: a comprehensive review; part 1. *Journal of Intensive Care Medicine*, (2), 163–175.

Seneff, M.G. (1987b) Central venous catheterisation: a comprehensive review; part 2. *Journal of Intensive Care Medicine*, (2), 218–232.

Sharma, A., Bodenham, A.R., & Mallick, A. (2004) Ultrasound-guided infraclavicular axillary vein cannulation for central venous access. *British Journal of Anaesthesia*, **93** (2), 188–192.

Stacey, R.G.W., Filshie, J. & Skewes, D. (1991) Percutaneous insertion of Hickman-type catheters. *British Journal of Hospital Medicine*, **46**, 396–398.

Tolar, B. & Gould, J.R. (1996) The timing and sequence of multiple device-related complications in patients with long-term indwelling Groshong catheters. *Cancer*, (78), 1308–1313.

Vesely, T.M. (2002) Optimal positioning of CVCs. *Journal of Vascular Access Devices*, **7** (3), 9–12.

Vesely, T.M. (2003) Central venous catheter tip position: a continuing controversy. *Journal of Cardiovascular and Interventional Radiology*, **14** (5), 527–534.

Weinstein, S.M. (2001) *Plumer's Principles and Practice of Infusion Therapy*, 7th edn. Lippincott, Williams & Wilkins, Philadelphia.

Winslow, M.N., Trammell, L. & Camp Sorrell, D. (1995) Selection of vascular access devices and nursing care. *Seminars in Oncology Nursing*, **11** (3), 167–173.

Wise, M., Richardson, D. & Lum, P. (2001) Catheter tip position: a sign of things to come. *Journal of Vascular Access Devices*, **6** (2), 18–27.

2 | Peripherally inserted central catheters (PICCs)

Peripherally inserted central catheters have made central venous access possible for many more patients due to their ease of insertion and the low complication rate associated with their use. The use of PICCs has increased rapidly and millions of PICCs are inserted every year. PICC placement is commonly undertaken by nurses in the USA where intravenous therapy is an integral part of their clinical practice (Gabriel 1996a). In the UK PICC insertion began in the mid 1990s, when nurses started to carry out placements in areas where they had previously been actively involved in peripheral cannulation: this was most common in the cancer setting.

LEARNING OBJECTIVES
By the end of this chapter the reader will be able to:

(1) Define a PICC.
(2) Identify the types available and their uses.
(3) Provide a description of the insertion procedure.
(4) Discuss immediate and follow-up care of the patient.
(5) Describe the removal process.

DEFINITION
Peripherally inserted central catheters are defined as catheters inserted via a peripheral vein and advanced along the upper arm to have the tip located in the lower third of the superior vena cava (NAVAN 1998; INS 2000; RCN 2003).

TYPES
PICCs can be made from silicone or polyurethane (see Fig. 2.1) (which usually contain a guidewire in order to provide the stiffness required for insertion). Most PICCs are configured

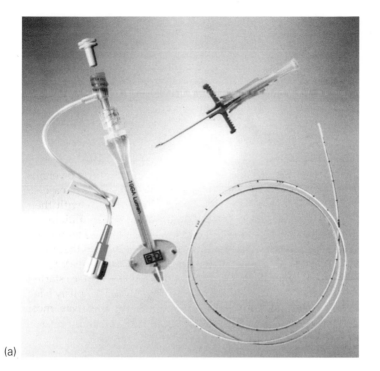

(a)

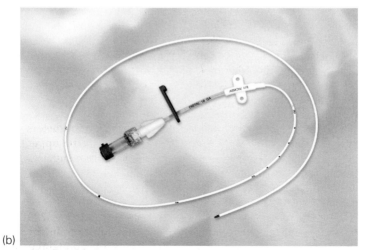

(b)

Fig. 2.1 (a) Silicone peripherally inserted central catheter (PICC), courtesy of Becton Dickinson. (b) Polyurethane PICC, courtesy of Arrow International, Inc.

Table 2.1 Average flow rates for PICCs.

Catheter	On gravity	On pump
4 Fr silicone	30–100 ml/hr	125–250 ml/hr
4 Fr polyurethane	66–187 ml/hr	545–965 ml/hr

as single or dual lumen, although triple lumen PICCs are now available for use in critical care patients (Costa & Ferguson 2002).

The lumen size varies depending on the material used. Silicone PICCs have smaller internal lumen, resulting in slow flow rates and higher potential for fragmentation if exposed to increased pressure injections. Polyurethane being the tougher material, enables thinner lumen walls and larger internal diameter of the lumens. This significantly increases flow rates and reduces the potential for breakage and rupture of the catheter (Mayer & Wong 2002). See Table 2.1. Sizing is usually referred to in French and the sizes range from 2–7 French.

They can measure from 50–70 cm in length. Some can be trimmed at the tip and others at the hub. Some of the polyurethane catheters have a silicone tip and can't be trimmed. The tips can be open-ended, valved at the tip or within the hub (see Fig. 1.4). There are some limitations on use: one is the use of CT contrast via a pressure injector. Williamson & McKinney (2001) studied the tolerance of silicone PICCs, in different sizes and lengths, to power injections of contrast materials at low rates suitable for CT scans. They found that the 3 Fr was unsuitable and could not accommodate flow rates; 4 Fr single and 6 Fr double withstood the flow, which was marginally adequate; 5 Fr single and 7 Fr tolerated peak flows and pressure well within the range. They were all shorter catheters, usually placed higher up the arm and the 35 cm length withstood higher flow rates than 45 cm, before failure. However, the MHRA (2004) issued a hazard warning regarding the use of all CVC and pressure injectors and recommended that CT contrast using a pressure injector was not injected through any CVAD.

INDICATIONS AND CONTRAINDICATIONS FOR PICC INSERTION
See Table 2.2.

USES OF PICCs IN VARIOUS SETTINGS

• In oncology: in patients with acute myeloid leukaemia it was shown that the PICC was an acceptable alternative long-term vascular access device (Strahilevitz et al. 2001). Snelling et al. (2001) compared PICCs with tunnelled catheters in patients with gastrointestinal cancers and found PICCs provided less invasive, more cost-effective and easier to book insertions when required for chemotherapy infusions. However, their

Table 2.2 Indications and contra-indications for PICC insertion.

Indications	Contra-indications
• Intermediate to long-term venous access • Patients requiring reliable venous access for short periods of time • Patients who have poor peripheral access in the lower arms • Patients in whom conventional central venous catheterisation may be hazardous, e.g. patients with low platelets, risk of pneumothorax, or who are vulnerable to infection • Patients requiring parenteral nutrition • Patients requiring repeated blood sampling (usually requires a catheter of 4 Fr and above) and for the administration of blood and blood products • Patient preference due to needle phobias, body image • Chest or neck sites unavailable or contra-indicated • Where tunnelled catheters are contra-indicated	• High volume fluid replacement • Compromised anatomy • Lymphoedema • Unable to identify or palpate antecubital veins (this may not be the case if ultrasound is available) • Previous recent infection or phlebitis • Lack of patient consent • Patient history of non-compliance with VADS • Lack of trained personnel to insert PICC • Patient wants to swim during therapy

(Adapted from Philpott & Griffiths 2003)

advantages over tunnelled catheters decreased significantly in treatment lasting longer than 120 days. Walshe et al. (2002) found a high complication rate but felt that the ease of insertion and removal argued for their use in cancer patients.

- In general medicine: Ng (1997) found PICCs could satisfy most long-term vascular needs and were safe in many patient populations. Infection rates did not depend on insertion mode, lumen number or patient's immune status. Arrowsmith (1999) found PICCs very useful in patients receiving TPN and recommended the PICC for therapies of 10–14 days.
- In critical care: Abi-Nader (1993) described clinical outcomes and cost for high risk critical care patients with PICCs in situ, and concluded that this was a safe alternative method to chest and neck insertion of central venous catheters. Griffiths & Philpot (2002) wished to determine if there was any significant difference between PICCs and central venous catheters in respect to length of stay of catheter, incidence of phlebitis and the need for removal due to infection. Results demonstrated that there was no significant difference in terms of gender, age and severity of illness. PICCs demonstrated a significantly longer length of stay and less phlebitis, and the authors concluded they could be used to provide a safe and effective alternative to non-tunnelled central venous catheters. They can also be used for CVP monitoring.

ADVANTAGES AND DISADVANTAGES OF PICCs

Advantages

- These catheters eliminate the risk associated with standard CVC placement both during insertion and once in situ. One of the greatest risks associated with any CVAD insertion is pneumothorax. This is highly unlikely to occur during PICC insertion, as the introducer needle is not placed near the lung. Those that have a guidewire within them are also safe, as the guidewire does not protrude from the catheter tip, is very fine and is made of a flexible material so that it cannot damage structures.

- Potential reduction of catheter-related bloodstream infections. There is evidence that shows that the use of PICCs is associated with a lower infection rate, although very few studies have been carried out comparing rates between PICCs and tunnelled catheters. Evidence appears to be related to the number of colony forming units (cfu) on the arm, compared with those present on the chest: the difference means that there is less cfu on the arm, which may help or reduce the risk of infection (Goodwin & Carlson 1993; Philpott & Griffiths 2003).
- Improved body image. For some patients, it is the body image aspect that makes the PICC a better option: there is very little risk of scarring either on insertion or removal, it does not result in a catheter exiting from the chest and can often be easily hidden under a sleeve. Gabriel (2003) found that patients were not troubled by the appearance of a PICC and that it had little impact on their lifestyle.
- Easy to use.
- Preservation of peripheral vascular system, avoids multiple venous cannulations (Philpott & Griffiths 2003).
- Reduction in discomfort and risk of dislodgement. By placing PICCs above the antecubital fossa, it has been shown to reduce movement of the catheter within the vein and therefore reduce the risk of phlebitis and thrombosis (Costa & Ferguson 2002).
- Reliability. It should be considered for vascular access of more than five days and Barbone (1995) concluded that if a PICC was carefully managed there was no reason why it could not remain in situ for up to 12 months (Gabriel 1996b; Philpott & Griffiths 2003).
- Sedation and surgical intervention (required for other CVADs) is not required.
- Preserves large vessels for more invasive therapies (Philpott & Griffiths 2003).

Disadvantages
One of the main disadvantages has been that patients required adequate access at the antecubital fossa in order to be able to have a PICC inserted. However, new technology has improved

access for patients by providing ultrasound imaging to enable the location of deeper veins in the upper arm, and this, along with a modified Seldinger technique (micropuncture or micro-introducer), has also improved the first time success rate. However, over time multiple insertions can cause venous scarring and decease the ability to reuse the site.

Another disadvantage is the difficulty patients have of redressing the site. Whereas other long-term CVAD do not require dressings, PICCs usually require a weekly dressing and this can be difficult to perform with one hand and so carers must be trained, or community staff involved. This can result in restrictions to the patient's lifestyle. There are also restrictions with bathing and swimming, although anecdotally it seems that patients indulge in other activities without restrictions.

Blood withdrawal can be difficult, depending on gauge size, and there is a tendency for PICCs to become sluggish more quickly than other CVADs when used for blood sampling. This is probably due to a build up of fibrin within the lumen, which slows down flow, particularly in silicone catheters. This is more noticeable in smaller catheters or if a dual lumen catheter is used.

Finally, malposition is a complication, either on insertion when the catheter may advance into a jugular, mammary or the contralateral subclavian vein, migrate into the jugular or be pulled back into the subclavian or axillary vein, resulting in an unsatisafactory tip location and risk of developing a thrombosis (Wise et al. 2001).

INSERTION

Insertion is carried out at the bedside and the insertion service in most hospitals has been nurse led. PICCs first came into use in the UK in the early 1990s. Gabriel published the first British article describing these devices and their uses in 1994, when nurses within oncology units started to gain training and supervision, and began to set up services. This was for a number of reasons, such as difficulty in getting access to other services for CVAD insertion (Alderman 1998), the need to provide patients with more choice, and the benefits and advantages that the device offered patients (Todd 1998, 2004). The developing service moved from oncology into other areas, such as parenteral nutrition and requirements for antibiotics in the community (Kayley 1999). Insertion is now carried out by many nurses in the UK and by some radiologists, where an interventional radiology service is available for difficult insertions.

Egan Sansivero (2001) highlighted that, historically, practitioners have utilised a landmark approach for CVAD insertion, and using anatomical landmarks for placement of PICCs certainly can result in successful placements, but that puncture-related complications are higher, especially the number of insertion attempts. Initial failures were referred to interventional radiology and this increased the success rates (Newman et al. 1998). Hand-held Doppler were used at the bedside and were inexpensive (MacRae 1998). Doppler has been highly effective in facilitating PICC placements (Gabriel 1999). In 1995 American radiologists demonstrated that ultrasound and fluoroscopy could be used for PICC placement. Using ultrasound and fluoroscopy often involves attendance at the radiology department, has financial implications and can delay treatment. However, success has been improved with use of a portable two-dimensional imaging machine used at the bedside, which resulted in less referrals to radiography. The use of two-dimensional ultrasound imaging is now recommended by NICE (2002) and can be used for a number of reasons (see Table 2.3).

Use of local anaesthetics
Due to the size of the introducer needle, patients should be offered local anaesthetic. This can be topical local anaesthetics which can be applied 30–60 minutes before the procedure or injectable local anaesthetic which tends to be used more when the microintroducer is used for insertion. Other methods are important to use in conjunction, such as use of relaxation techniques; distraction and anxiolytics (Moureau & Zonderman 2000). Bahruth (1996) found that the use of local anaesthetic (EMLA™) resulted in significant vasoconstriction and/or venospasm in all of the patients in the sample, which resulted in difficult insertions in those patients, and also affected advancement of the catheter. These problems did not occur in those who did not have any local anaesthetic.

Table 2.3 Use of ultrasound.

- Allows the visualisation of the size of the median cubital, basilic, cephalic, and brachial veins so that the practitioner can choose the appropriate size catheter. This, in turn, will reduce the potential risk of post-insertion complications, such as thrombosis and phlebitis.

- Allows visualisation of the patency of the vein selected. This can then reduce the incidence of post-insertion complications and reduce possible problems with the advancement of the catheter along the patient's arm.

- Allows visualisation of the location of peripheral veins and arterial structures in order to reduce the risk of an arterial puncture or the number of attempts at venous punctures.

- Enables the placement of a PICC in the upper arm. This can reduce the risk of damage to the catheter due to arm movement.

- Enables the placement of a dual lumen catheter, when required, instead of the patient having to settle for a single lumen catheter that can only be inserted using palpation, direct visualisation or anatomical landmarks.

(Adapted from Kokotis 2001)

Preparation for insertion – choosing a vein

Patients are not required to starve and, unless very anxious, no sedation is required. The patient is then laid prone and an assessment of the veins is performed to ascertain which vein is most suitable.

Veins used for PICC insertion are usually as follows (Fig. 1.1):

- The median basilic vein is the first choice of vein, due to its size and because it offers the shortest and straightest route to the subclavian. It has fewer valves than the other veins and fewer junctions to negotiate. It is 8 mm in diameter and 24 cm long (NAVAN 1998).
- The median cubital is a large and well-supported vein, but tends to have junctions low in the antecubital fossa, which can result in problems with advancing. However, it is a large and easily accessible vein and so is the second choice.
- The median cephalic is large but then narrows just above the antecubital fossa (6 mm), has many valves within it and

also results in the catheter having to negotiate a turn as it advances from the axillary vein into the subclavian vein. This often results in problems with advancement (McPhee 1999; Perucca 2001).

Left side or right side placement?

Many patients who are right-handed prefer to have their PICC placed in the left arm. This can cause problems for the inserting practitioner as it has a longer course to travel, the tip may not advance easily into the vena cava and it can butt up against the wall of the brachiocephalic vein, resulting in trauma and difficulty bleeding the device. Right-sided placement offers a shorter route with a more direct approach into the vena cava. Whichever arm is used it must be remembered that there is a tendency for the PICC tip to move in a caudal direction with the change in arm position from abduction to adduction. Up to 58% of PICCs move 20 mm or more and this change in position should be considered during final catheter tip positioning (Forauer & Alonzo 2000).

Measurement of catheter

There are various methods for measuring patients to ensure that the PICC is inserted the correct distance to enable the tip to be located correctly and this may be in order to cut the catheter prior to insertion (open-ended catheters) or on completion (valved catheters). Initially, measurement was performed by measuring from the intended venepuncture site to the top of the shoulder, adding the length of the clavicle and finally the measurement to the third intercostal space. This did not always prove accurate. Lum (1999) developed a slightly different method, where the measurement was taken with the arm at 45° and measured from the venepuncture site diagonally to the middle of the clavicle. Then the length of the clavicle was added for right-sided placements, and for left-sided the width of the manubrium was added (about 2–4 cm) (See Fig. 2.2). Now, Lum (2004) has developed a formula-based measurement guide based on patient height, to ensure optimal tip positioning and found that 97% of the total 382 insertions were successfully placed with the CVC tip in the distal SVC. He concluded that the tailored-fit formula to individual height is a reliable tool to predict CVC length (see Table 2.4).

Positioning of patient

Once the catheter has been advanced a short way up the arm (about 20 cm) the arm can be moved to a right angle to enable a straight route, and the head is turned towards the arm of insertion, with the chin tucked down on the clavicle. This position helps to reduce the risk of advancing the catheter up along the jugular vein. The practitioner can gauge when there are

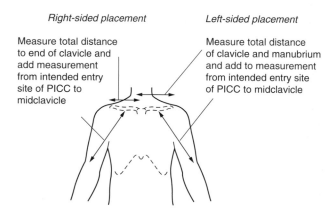

Right-sided placement

Measure total distance to end of clavicle and add measurement from intended entry site of PICC to midclavicle

Left-sided placement

Measure total distance of clavicle and manubrium and add to measurement from intended entry site of PICC to midclavicle

Fig. 2.2 Pre-insertion measurement of a PICC.

Table 2.4 Lum (2004) formula for measurement guide for optimal positioning of catheter tip.

Right PICC = 3 × height of patient divided by 10
  e.g. (3 × 152 cm) ÷ 10 = 45.6 cm
Left PICC = 3 × patient's height divided by 10 + 4 cm
  e.g. [(3 × 152 cm) ÷ 10] + 4 cm = 49.6 cm
These measurements are based on the standard PICC site being approximately 2.5 cm below the antecubital fossa.

---

problems with placement by asking the patient during insertion if they have any aural sensations; this has been described as a whooshing or gurgling sound behind the ear. This could indicate that the tip is along the jugular vein and that any flushing solution will then be heard behind the ear. However, tip placement is always verified following insertion, by a chest X-ray, which should be done immediately after insertion and before infusion via the device (Royer 2001). Problems with advancement of the catheter and malposition of the catheter tip can occur for a variety of reasons, and conditions such as a mediastinal mass can increase the risk of catheter malposition (Tamburro et al. 2003). Therefore, it is important to assess the patient carefully and obtain a detailed history prior to insertion. An overview of the procedure is described in Table 2.5.

Problems that may occur during insertion
There may be difficulty in advancing due to:

- Incorrect positioning of the patient; ask the patient to gently rotate the wrist and relax the shoulder to allow for easy advancement.
- Venospasm: force should not be used to advance the catheter. If the vein is in spasm, apply a warm compress to dilate the vein. Use slow strokes when advancing to prevent spasm.
- Valves: flushing as the catheter is advanced can help to open the valves. Patient can open and close hand to help open the valves.
- Malposition: if the catheter is kinked within the vein or advancing up an axillary vein then it may prevent advancement. Checks can be made with ultrasound during the procedure. However, if the catheter kinks at insertion site it should be removed.

IMMEDIATE CARE
Securement and dressing of the device is vital. PICCs are designed so that they can be sutured. However, suture securement relies on integrity of the skin and this site can became inflamed and lead to bacterial colonisation of the exit site (Schears 2005). Therefore, suturing is not recommended

Table 2.5 Insertion of a PICC.

(1) Patient is positioned lying flat, arms at side.
(2) If topical LA cream has been applied, it is wiped off and a tourniquet applied.
(3) A measurement is performed (see Fig. 2.3).
(4) The practitioner scrubs up, whilst the assistant opens the packs.
(5) The practitioner puts on a sterile gown and sterile gloves and prepares the packs and the catheter (e.g. flushing to check patency and cutting to correct length where necessary).
(6) The practitioner then cleans the patient's skin and drapes the patient with a fenestrated drape.
(7) The tourniquet is tightened and the practitioner removes gloves and puts on a fresh sterile pair.
(8) The introducer needle is inserted into the vein (or a cannula inserted, a guidewire passed, small incision made following infiltration of local anaesthetic and a dilator introducer passed) and the tourniquet is released.
(9) Digital pressure is applied above the introducer and the needle removed and disposed of into a sharps container.
(10) The catheter is then inserted into the introducer and advanced along the vein.
(11) At a certain point the patient will be asked to move their arm to a right angle and turn their head towards the practitioner, tucking their chin down onto their clavicle (to prevent advancing the catheter along the jugular vein).
(12) During advancement the catheter is flushed and checked for blood return, at regular intervals.
(13) Once the catheter has been advanced to the designated length, where appropriate, the guidewire is removed and the introducer is withdrawn, split and peeled off the catheter.
(14) The catheter is then flushed to check for patency.
(15) Finally, a securing device is applied and the insertion site is covered with a transparent dressing.

(Hanchett 1999; Maki 2002). Securement is usually by the use of sterile strips such as Steristrips™ and/or a specifically designed securing device such as a Statlock™ (see Fig. 2.3). This will help to reduce mechanical phlebitis, catheter migration, catheter damage and granuloma (Gabriel 2001; Crnich & Maki 2002; Yamamoto et al. 2002; Schears 2005). The dressing at the site should allow visual inspection and provide sterility, as well as reducing the risk of infection. The recommended dressing is a

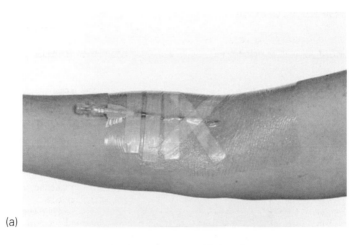

(a)

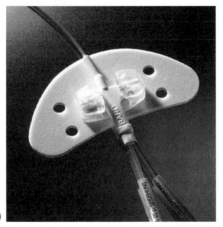

(b)

Fig. 2.3 Securement using (a) Steristrips™ (Finlay 2004), (b) the adhesive securement dressing Statlock™ (part (b) courtesy of Venetec International, Inc.).

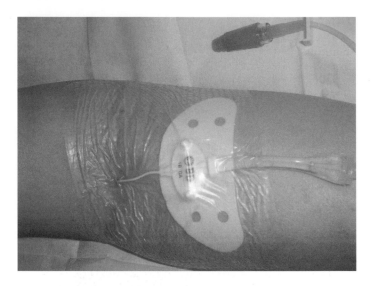

Fig. 2.4 PICC insertion site dressed using a transparent dressing.

transparent semi-permeable dressing, which allows moisture permeability (DoH 2001; NICE 2003; RCN 2003) (see Fig. 2.4). Bleeding occurs within the first 24 hours, so a small fold of sterile gauze should be placed over the site and under the dressing (Philpott & Griffiths 2003). The device should be flushed with 0.9% sodium chloride, and then, where appropriate (usually with open-ended catheters), a heparinised saline solution, e.g. Hepsal™ (10 iu of heparin in 1 ml sodium chloride, usual dose of 50 iu/5 ml) to maintain patency (DoH 2001; NICE 2003; RCN 2003).

FOLLOW-UP CARE

Patients may complain of an aching sensation in the upper arm in the first 24–48 hours following insertion. This is usually caused by mechanical phlebitis and can be resolved by using a warm pack over the area and resting the limb. If this has not resolved within 72–96 hours it may necessitate the removal of the PICC.

The initial dressing should be changed after 24 hours (Ryder 2001) and thereafter the dressing and flushing of the PICC should be carried out weekly (RCN 2003). The site should be inspected for any signs of infection and/or phlebitis. The dressing should be changed more frequently if it is found to be loose or contaminated at all. Patients should be supplied with written information and adequate supplies of cleaning solutions, dressings, etc. (see Chapter 9).

REMOVAL

Removal of a PICC is relatively straightforward; the patient does not need to lie flat and once the dressing has been removed, gentle traction on the catheter will allow removal. The nurse should check the integrity of the catheter and check the measurement of the catheter against the original length inserted. If this does not correspond they should inform a doctor as this may indicate a catheter embolism. If the catheter is removed due to a suspected or confirmed infection the tip should be cut off and sent to the microbiology laboratory for culturing.

Marx (1995) found that as PICCs lie wholly within the venous system, except for a short course though skin and subcutaneous tissue, they can usually be removed with slow gentle traction. Venous spasm is more likely in those who have had the catheter inserted for a short time frame (less than 15 days), if there has been chemical or mechanical irritation, valve inflammation, or the patient has fears and anxieties. If there is phlebitis this may be associated with venous spasm and cause removal of a PICC to be uncomfortable or painful. Firm, constant, but gentle traction may overcome mild venous resistance or spasm. Care must be taken not to damage the catheter. In this case the pressure should be released and removal attempted again after a 30-minute rest.

During this time the following can also be tried:

- Give the patient a warm drink.
- Apply a warm compress.
- Administer a warm saline infusion.
- Attempt mental distraction and relaxation.

Removal can then be reattempted. If there is still a problem, a doctor should be informed and it may be necessary to wait

12–24 hours. If a fibrin sheath or thrombus is well organised a surgical cutdown may be required to remove it. Difficulty may occur in 1% of removals (Drewett 2000).

Scenario

Mrs Smith, a 45-year-old patient with cancer of the ovary, has had a peripherally inserted central catheter in situ for two months. Initially, she had phlebitis for four days after insertion, with some erythema and swelling. She has now presented at the day unit with swelling of the whole upper arm with the PICC in, and pain along the arm and into the shoulder and neck. She also tells you that four days ago the catheter got pulled and she thinks it is a bit longer.

What will you do, and what do you suspect is the cause of her symptoms?

When the dressing is taken down, it is found that the catheter has moved out 10 cm and on X-ray the tip is now lying in the subclavian vein. On ultrasound it is discovered that a thrombus has formed around the catheter. This is causing the pain and swelling. This may have occurred as the tip was not in the correct position and made Mrs Smith more susceptible to thrombosis. The PICC is removed and Mrs Smith is commenced on a heparin infusion.

CONCLUSION

PICCs are a relatively straightforward catheter to insert, with few hazards, which makes it a suitable device for any vulnerable patients. Their ease of use has enabled greater accessibility for patients, as nurses develop more PICC services, which in itself has also increased the settings in which patients can now receive their treatment.

REFERENCES

Abi-Nader, J.A. (1993) Peripherally inserted central venous catheters in critical care patients. *Heart and Lung*, (22), 428–434.

Alderman, C. (1998) Chemo by catheter. *Nursing Standard*, **12** (28), 25–27.

Arrowsmith, H. (1999) Case study approach to PICCs. *British Journal of Nursing*, **8** (18), 1231–1238.

Bahruth, A.J. (1996) PICC insertion problems associated with topical anaesthetic. *Journal of Intravenous Nursing*, **19** (1), 32–34.

Barbone, M. (1995) Vascular access device patency. Paper presented at the 9th National Association of Vascular Access Networks conference, Salt Lake City, Utah (Sept.) and cited by Gabriel, J. (1996a) Care and management of PICCs. *British Journal of Nursing*, **5** (10), 594–599.

Costa, N. & Ferguson, E. (2002) Placement of triple lumen – peripherally inserted central catheters in critical patients. *Journal of Vascular Access Devices*, **7** (4), 27–32.

Crnich, C.J. & Maki, D.G. (2002) The promise of novel technology for the prevention of intravascular device-related bloodstream infections; part 2. Long-term devices, healthcare epidemiology. *Clinical Infectious Diseases*, **34** (10), 1362–1368.

Department of Health (2001) Guidelines for preventing infections associated with the insertion and maintenance of central venous catheters. *Journal of Hospital Infection*, **47** (supplement), S47–S67.

Drewett, S. (2000) Central venous catheter removal: procedures and rationale. *British Journal of Nursing*, **9** (22), 2304–2315.

Egan Sansivero, G. (2001) Use of imaging and microintroducer technology. *Journal of Vascular Access Devices*, **6** (1), 7–13.

Forauer, A.R. & Alonzo, M. (2000) Change in peripherally inserted central catheter tip position with abduction and adduction of the upper extremity. *Journal of Vascular and Interventional Radiology*, (11), 1315–1318.

Finlay, T. (2004) *Intravenous Therapy.* Blackwell Publishing, Oxford.

Gabriel, J. (1994) An intravenous alternative. *Nursing Times*, **90** (31), 39–41.

Gabriel, J. (1996a) Care and management of PICCs. *British Journal of Nursing*, **5** (10), 594–599.

Gabriel, J. (1996b) PICC expanding UK nurses' practice. *British Journal of Nursing*, **5** (2), 71–74.

Gabriel, J. (1999) PICCs: how Doppler ultrasound can extend their use. *Nursing Times*, **95** (6), 52–53.

Gabriel, J. (2001) PICC securement: minimise potential complications. *Nursing Standard*, **15** (43), 42–44.

Gabriel, J. (2003) Peripherally inserted central catheters: patient involvement. *Cancer Nursing Practice*, **2** (8), 27–32.

Goodwin, M. & Carlson, I. (1993) The peripherally inserted central catheter: a retrospective look at three years of insertions. *Journal of Intravenous Nursing*, **16** (2), 92–103.

Griffiths, V.R. & Philpott, P. (2002) PICCs: do they have a role in the care of the critically ill patient? *Intensive and Critical Care Nursing*, **18**, 37–47.

Hanchett, M. (1999) Science of intravenous securement. *Journal of Vascular Access Devices*, **4** (3), 9–15.

Intravenous Nursing Society (INS) (2000) *Standards for Infusion Therapy.* Beckon Dickinson and Intravenous Nursing Society, Massachusetts, USA.

Kayley, J. (1999) Intravenous therapy in the community. In: Dougherty, L. & Lamb, J. (eds) *Intravenous Therapy in Nursing Practice*. Churchill Livingstone, Edinburgh.

Kokotis, K. (2001) New trends in vascular access therapy. *Journal of Vascular Access Devices*, (Summer), 7–10.

Lum, P. (1999) Techniques for optimising tip position. Presentation at National Association of Vascular Access Networks 13th Annual Conference, Orlando.

Lum, P. (2004) A new formula-based measurement guide for optimal positioning of central venous catheters. *Journal of Association of Vascular Access*, **9** (2), 80–85.

MacRae, K. (1998) Hand-held Dopplers in central catheter insertion. *Professional Nurse*, **14** (2), 99–102.

Maki, D.G. (2002) The promise of novel technology for prevention of intravascular device related bloodstream infections. National Association of Vascular Access Networks conference presentation (Sept.). San Diego.

Marx, M. (1995) The management of the difficult peripherally inserted central venous catheter line removal. *Journal of Intravenous Nursing*, **18** (5), 246–249.

Mayer, T. & Wong, D.G. (2002) The use of polyurethane PICCs: an alternative to other materials. *Journal of Vascular Access Devices*, (Summer), 26–29.

McPhee, A. (1999) *Handbook of Infusion Therapy.* Springhouse Corporation, Pennsylvania.

Medicines and Healthcare Products Regulatory Agency (MHRA) (2004) *Risk of Catheter Rupture During Contrast CT Investigation Due to Over Pressurisation When Used With a Power Injector.* MDA/2004/010 (25, February) Medicines and Healthcare Products Regulatory Agency, London. www.mhra.gov.uk

Moureau, N. & Zonderman, A. (2000) Does it always have to hurt? *Journal of Intravenous Nursing*, **23** (4), 213–219.

National Institute for Clinical Excellence (NICE) (2002) *Ultrasound imaging for central venous catheter placement*. Department of Health, London.

National Institute for Clinical Excellence (NICE) (2003) *Infection Control Prevention of Healthcare Associated Infection in Primary and*

Community Care, Clinical Guidelines 2. Department of Health, London.

National Association of Vascular Access Networks (1998) Tip location of peripherally inserted central catheters. *Journal of Vascular Access Devices*, **8** (Summer).

Newman, M.L., Murphy, B.D. & Rosen, M.P. (1998) Bedside placement of PICCs: a cost-effectiveness analysis. *Radiology*, (206), 423–428.

Ng, P.K., Ault, M.J., Gray Elrodt, A. & Maldonado, L. (1997) PICC in general medicine. *Mayo Clinic Proceedings*. No. 72, 225–233.

Perucca, R. (2001) Obtaining vascular access. In: Carlson, K., Perdue, M.B. & Hankins, J. (eds) *Infusion Therapy in Clinical Practice*, 2nd edn. W.B. Saunders, Pennsylvania.

Philpott, P. & Griffiths, V.R. (2003) The peripherally inserted central catheter. *Nursing Standard*, **17** (44), 39–46.

Royal College of Nursing Intravenous Therapy Forum (2003) *RCN Standards for Infusion Therapy*. Royal College of Nursing, London.

Royer, T. (2001) A case for posterior, anterior, and lateral chest X-rays being performed following each PICC placement. *Journal of Vascular Access Devices*, **6** (4), 9–11.

Ryder, M. (2001) The role in biofilm in vascular catheter related infections. *New Developments in Vascular Diseases*, **2** (2), 15–25.

Schears, G.J. (2005) The benefits of a catheter securement device on reducing patient complications. *Managing Hospital Infection*, **5** (2), 14–20.

Snelling, R., Jones, G., Figueredo, A. & Major, I. (2001) Central venous catheters for infusion therapy in gastrointestinal cancer. *Journal of Intravenous Nursing*, **24** (1), 38–47.

Strahilevitz, J., Lossos, I.S., Verstandig, A., Sasson, T., Kori, Y. & Gillis, S. (2001) Vascular access via peripherally inserted central venous catheters experience in 40 patients with AML at a single institute. *Leukemia and Lymphoma*, **40** (3–4), 365–371.

Tamburro, R.F. (2003) The effect of a mediastinal mass on the initial positioning of a PICC. *Journal of Intravenous Nursing*, **26** (3), 92–96.

Todd, J. (1998) Peripherally inserted central catheters. *Professional Nurse*, **13** (5), 297–302.

Todd, J. (2004) Choice and use of peripherally inserted central catheters by nurses. *Professional Nurse*, **19** (9), 493–497.

Walshe, L.J., Malak, S.F., Eagan, J. & Sepkowits, K.A. (2002) Complication rates among cancer patients with peripherally inserted central catheters. *Journal of Clinical Oncology*, **20** (15), 3276–3281.

Williamson, E.E. & McKinney, J.M. (2001) Assessing the adequacy of PICC for power injection of intravenous contrast agents for CT. *Journal of Computer Assisted Tomography*, **25** (6), 932–937.

Wise, M., Richardson, D. & Lum, P. (2001) Catheter tip position: a sign of things to come. *Journal of Vascular Access Devices*, **6** (2), 18–27.

Yamamoto, A.J., Solomon, J.A., Soulen, M.C., Tang, J., Parkinson, K., Lin, R. & Schears, G.J. (2002) Sutureless securement devices reduce the complications of peripherally inserted central venous catheters. *Journal of Vascular and Interventional Radiology*, **13** (1), 77–81.

Non-tunnelled short-term central venous catheters $\quad$ 3

These catheters have been used for many years. Seneff (1987a) wrote that the central venous catheter (CVC) is an indispensable technique in today's practice of medicine. It was initially used to monitor central venous pressure but it is now more commonly established to administer intravenous drugs. The first description of subclavian venepuncture in humans was in 1952. A major advance in intravenous catheter techniques came when, in 1953, Seldinger described the catheter placement over a needle using a guidewire, a technique that now bears his name. In 1957 the clinical use of central venous pressure measurement in humans was developed.

LEARNING OBJECTIVES
By the end of this chapter the reader will be able to:

(1) List the uses for a non-tunnelled CVC.
(2) Discuss the advantages and disadvantages.
(3) Provide a description of the insertion procedure.
(4) Discuss immediate and follow-up care of the patient.
(5) Describe the removal process.
(6) Show an understanding of the principles of CVP monitoring.

DEFINITION
A non-tunnelled central venous catheter is a catheter inserted directly into the vein with its tip usually located in the vena cava or right atrium.

TYPES
Most catheters are made of polyurethane, and are comprised of multiple lumens: three, four or five (see Fig. 3.1). They are provided in varying lengths and French sizes. The tips are

open-ended, either at the end of the catheter tip or staggered along the length of the catheter.

USES

This catheter is used mainly for emergency access, in the theatre and critical care setting and where short-term central venous access is required.

Advantages

- It is quick to insert, making it useful in emergency and critical care settings.
- Its multi-lumen access makes it useful for multiple therapies.
- Can be used for central venous pressure and haemodynamic monitoring.

Disadvantages

There are many disadvantages to using this catheter. The fact that it is used in an emergency exposes the patients to the

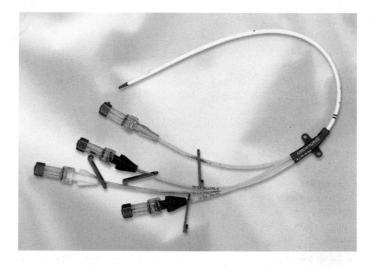

Fig. 3.1 Example of a multi-lumen CVC (courtesy of Arrow International, Inc.).

commonest complication, which is the risk of pneumothorax and haemorrhage as the needle punctures the vein directly above major organs (such as the lung) and vessels (such as the carotid artery). The other risk associated with this catheter is infection. Again, the direct entry into the vein results in an increased risk of infection, as the bacteria can track along the catheter from the insertion site. This has resulted in the development of catheters that are impregnated with anti-bactericidals, antiseptics and antibiotics. These can be applied to the outer lumen or may be present within the lumen itself. It has been shown that these are particularly useful in reducing the risk of a gram-positive infection staphylococcus aureus. The DoH (2001) recommended that these catheters be used within high-risk areas, such as critical care and oncology. Problems are the possible development of antibiotic resistance, cost implications (as they are more expensive than conventional catheters) and the lack of efficacy against gram-negative infections (see Chapter 7 for more details).

INSERTION

Medical staff usually perform the insertion of central venous catheters; however, in some areas nurses are developing a role in inserting these devices. There are a number of key aspects for aiding the inserting practitioner that the nurse can perform:

(1) Preparing the patient for the procedure.
(2) Positioning of the patient, and raising and tilting the bed.
(3) Teaching the patient about the Valsalva manoeuvre.

The Valsalva manoeuvre may be performed by conscious patients to aid the insertion of a CVC. The patient is placed in the Trendelenberg position. They are asked to breath in and try to force the air, with the mouth closed and nose pinched closed (i.e. against a closed glottis). This increases the intra-thoracic pressure from a normal 3–4 mmHg to 60–70 mmHg, so that the return of blood to the heart is momentarily reduced and as a result the veins in the neck region become engorged (McPhee 1999). Ostrow (1981) suggests that a venous distension of up to 2.5 cm can be achieved using this manoeuvre (Scales 1999; Hatchett 2000; Weinstein 2001; Dougherty 2004).

Vein selection

There are a number of veins commonly used for the insertion of CVC (Table 3.1). There are no absolute contraindications to central venous catheterisation in patients who require it, but there may be contra-indications to specific approaches (Seneff 1987a). The ipsilateral limb associated with lymph node dissection or radical neck dissection should be avoided, as there is limited tissue in the supraclavicular area, making a catheter tract prominent. Concurrent radiation to the site could impede wound healing. Prediction of procedural risk in patients with severe thrombocytopenia will enable the transfusion of platelets. Concurrent anticoagulant and administration of antiplatelet agents should be stopped temporarily. Patients with fibrinogen deficiency/liver dysfunction may require FFP and/or vitamin K prior to insertion (Egan Sansivero 1998).

Table 3.1 Insertion sites, possible complications and management problems.

Subclavian	Moderate complication risk. Pneumothorax and thoracic duct injury are increased risks in this area.	Problems with shoulder movement if sutured laterally. Contamination by tracheal or oral secretions.
Jugular	Moderate complications. Brachial plexus injury. Thrombosis.	Difficult dressing applications. Neck movement loosens dressing. Contamination by hair, tracheal or oral secretions.
Femoral	Lower complication risk. Highest risk of sepsis, thrombosis and immobility complications.	Site easily contaminated by urine and faeces. Difficult to place and maintain dressing due to movement.

(Reproduced with permission of Elsevier from Evans Orr 1993)

Common veins are:

- subclavian;
- external and internal jugular;
- femoral.

External jugular

This is the primary site for central venous catheterisation in patients who are anticoagulated and is the alternative site to the internal jugular for those who cannot tolerate even a small pneumothorax. The advantages of this route are that it is part of the surface anatomy, observable, easily entered and can be cannulated in the presence of clotting abnormalities. The risk of pneumothorax is also avoided (Seneff 1987a; Scales 1999; Weinstein 2001).

Internal jugular

This vein is a good site for central venous catheterisation as it is associated with a high success rate and low incidence of complications. There is a risk of carotid puncture (this constitutes 80–95% of all complications), and laceration of neck structures with a probing needle, unless ultrasound is used. There is also less morbidity, thrombosis and stenosis (Seneff 1987b).

Subclavian

The puncture of this vein is quick and easy to learn and uses identifiable and consistent landmarks. Once inserted, the catheter is comfortable for patients and easy to maintain on a long-term basis. Complications include pneumothorax and malposition (Seneff 1987b).

Femoral

This is the easiest of all central venous procedures to learn and perform. The anatomy is predictable; recognisable landmarks usually present and the vein is large. Long-term cannulation of the femoral vein should be avoided, but short-term (24 hours) is useful. It is associated with minor risks at the time of venepuncture and may be performed during CPR without stopping chest compressions (Seneff 1987a).

Inferior vena cava

The translumbar and transhepatic approach is usually reserved for patients with stenosis and/or thrombosis of SVC (Seneff 1987b).

Technique

There are three methods of central venous placement:

- Over a needle: this method involves the use of an extra long cannula and is most commonly associated with placement of cannulae in the internal jugular vein (Scales 1999).
- Through a cannula: this technique uses a small wide-bore cannula, which is inserted into a central vein and is used for the placement of transvenous pacing wires (Scales 1999).
- Over a guidewire: this method of placement is known as the Seldinger technique. The vein is punctured using a needle, a guidewire is then passed and the needle withdrawn. This is the procedure described below (Scales 1999) (see Fig. 3.2).

The patient should be placed in 15–30° Trendelenberg position, arms to side and head turned to contralateral side. The Valsalva manoeuvre should be used in conscious patients, to distend the veins in dehydrated patients and to aid in identification of the vessel. Once the vessel is located, using a large bore needle attached to a syringe or cannula, venepuncture is performed using the index finger and thumb to distend and anchor the vein. Blood flashback confirms the placement of the cannula in the blood vessel. The syringe is removed and a guidewire is inserted through the cannula. The use of a J-wire improves efficiency as the J shape to the end facilitates its passage around corners (Scales 1999). The cannula is then removed and the guidewire is advanced into the vessel. A dilator is used to dilate the blood vessel and a small incision is made to ensure the catheter can be advanced. The catheter is advanced over the guidewire, which is then removed. The catheter is advanced to a maximum of 15 cm in a right-sided jugular or subclavian insertion and in smaller adults, and 20–30 cm for left-sided subclavian and larger adults (Baranowski 1993).

The Seldinger technique can be used when inserting a central venous catheter over a guide wire. These illustrations show the step-by-step process of the Seldinger technique.

Locate the vein to be cannulated. Then insert a small (18G) needle into the vein.

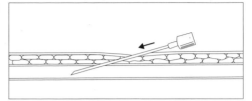

Pass the guide wire through the needle, and thread it into the vein.

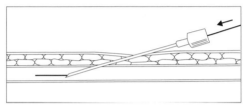

With the guide wire remaining in place, withdraw the needle.

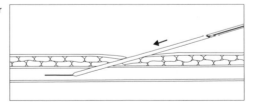

Advance the catheter over the guide wire into the vein. Rotate the catheter as you advance it over the guide wire.

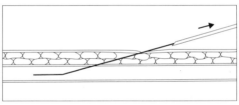

With the catheter in place, carefully re-move the guide wire.

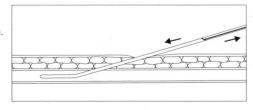

Fig. 3.2 Insertion of a CVC using the Seldinger technique. Redrawn from McPhee, A. (1999) *Handbook of Infusion Therapy* with permission of Lippincott Williams & Wilkins.

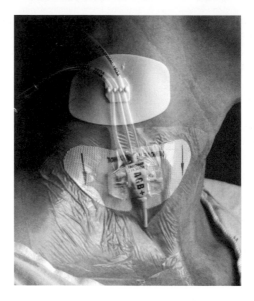

Fig. 3.3 Securing device for a CVC (courtesy of Venetec International, Inc.).

IMMEDIATE CARE

The catheter may be sutured into place, but recent recommendations are to secure the catheter with a specially designed securement device, such as those illustrated in Fig. 3.3. This is because of the risk of infection associated with sutures (Crnich & Maki 2002; Maki 2005). Once the catheter has been secured it should be covered with a transparent sterile dressing. Gauze may be applied over the site initially, to soak up any exudate, but the dressing and the gauze should be removed after 24 hours, the site inspected and a new transparent dressing applied. A chest X-ray should be carried out and the tip location documented in the patient's notes.

FOLLOW-UP CARE

The dressing can then be changed once or twice a week, or whenever necessary. One of the biggest difficulties with non-tunnelled catheters is that they are often placed in the jugular vein and this makes dressing very awkward. The catheter hangs down, pulling on the dressing, exposing the site to contamination, and can be uncomfortable for the patient. This is further hindered in men as their beard grows and the dressing does not adhere to the skin. This is also a problem in patients who are febrile or sweaty.

REMOVAL

Whilst the removal of a CVC can appear to be straightforward it is not without complications, the main risk being an air embolism. See Table 3.2. for the correct procedure to follow. The patients should be placed in the Trendelenberg position, head

Table 3.2 Procedure for removal.

(1) Explain the procedure to the patient and give instructions related to the Valsalva maneouvre.
(2) Discontinue any therapy in progress.
(3) Gather the required equipment and place on a trolley.
(4) Position the patient in the Trendelenberg position.
(5) Wash hands with bactericidal soap and water or bactericidal alcohol handrub.
(6) Open sterile pack and empty all contents onto the pack.
(7) Wash hands with bactericidal alcohol handrub.
(8) Loosen old dressing.
(9) Put on clean gloves and remove the old dressing and discard.
(10) If the site is red or discharging then take a swab.
(11) Remove gloves and put on sterile gloves.
(12) Clean the insertion site.
(13) Clean the gloves with bactericidal alcohol handrub.
(14) Cut and remove any skin sutures securing the catheter or remove the securing device.
(15) Ask the patient to perform the Valsalva manoeuvre.
(16) Place a sterile swab over the insertion site and as the catheter is removed, using slow and steady traction, apply pressure.
(17) Maintain pressure on the swab for about five minutes.
(18) If the catheter has been removed due to infection then ensure the catheter tip is cut using sterile scissors and placed in a sterile container.
(19) When the bleeding has stopped cover the site with a waterproof transparent dressing to prevent air entry via the insertion site.
(20) Where necessary send the tip and swab to the laboratory for microbiological investigation.
(21) Discard all waste appropriately.

lower than feet so that the risk of any air entry is reduced. This, coupled with the patient performing the Valsalva manoeuvre during removal, will reduce the chances of air embolus. A transparent occlusive dressing is recommended and should remain in place for at least 24 hours (Scales 1999) (see Chapter 7).

CENTRAL VENOUS PRESSURE MONITORING

Measuring central venous pressure (CVP)

CVP is the pressure of blood in the right atrium of the heart and vena cava. It provides information about the following (Higgins 2004):

- blood volume in relation to current capacity;
- vascular tone;
- effectiveness of right-sided cardiac function;
- pulmonary vascular resistance;
- intra-thoracic pressure.

Measurements can be carried out using different equipment depending on the setting (Manley 1991; Woodrow 1992; Henderson 1997; *Nursing Standard* 1999; Weinstein 2001; Brighton 2004) (Table 3.3):

(1) General ward: CVP is measured in cm H_2O in a column, with the zero point being level with the patient's right atrium. This is known as the water manometer system (Higgins 2004).
(2) Critical care units: pressure transducer, needs pressure monitoring equipment.

The normal values range from 3–15 cm water (3–10 mmHg) (Higgins 2004). A CVP can be expected to rise by 5 cm (2 mmHg) when patients are intubated and artificially ventilated using intermittent positive pressure ventilation (Gourley 1996; Hatchett 2000; Brighton 2004).

Measurements can be taken at two points: sternal angle and mid-axilla point (see Fig. 3.4). Several readings are necessary to indicate a response, as single readings are of little use. A combination of place and patient position must be recorded, so that all

Table 3.3 Procedure for monitoring central venous pressure.

(1) Explain the procedure to the patient.
(2) Check the device is patent with a saline flush.
(3) CVP measurements can be taken from the mid-axilla so that the baseline of the manometer is in line with the right atrium. A variety of positions are suited to using the mid-axilla as a point of reference. Ideally, the patient should be in a semi-recumbent or recumbent position. Record the position of the patient.
(4) If the patient is supine an alternative position is via the sternal angle. It is important to choose one method and mark the site, after gaining the patient's permission. Record the site in the nursing notes. Readings from the sternal angle are about 5 cm lower than those taken from mid-axilla.
(5) Adjust the manometer scale so the baseline figure 0 is lined up with zero on the arm of the spirit level.
(6) Check that the baseline and right atrium are level by extending the arm of the spirit level to the sternal angle or mid-axilla. Move the manometer scale until the bubble is between the parallel lines on the spirit level.
(7) Turn the three-way tap to the patient (see Fig. 3.5). Allow the manometer to fill slowly with fluid from the infusion bag. Do not overfill manometer. Turn off the three-way tap to the intravenous fluids; the column of fluid in the manometer should fill rapidly.
(8) When the level of fluid in the manometer ceases to drop, starting to rise and fall with the patient's respiration, the reading can be taken.
(9) Reading may be taken from the top (8.5) or below (6) of the oscillating fluid level. Turn off the three-way tap to the manometer and readjust infusion rates.

There are other methods, but the same method should be used each time to ensure consistency.

subjective measurements can be taken at the same place and provide consistent measurements. Central venous pressure measurement is useful in measuring blood and fluid replacement as well as acute cardiovascular failure and unstable cardiovascular dynamic states, oliguria and anuria (Gourley 1996).

The following should be considered when there are changes in the reading (Table 3.4):

(1) Have all measurements been performed in a consistent way?
(2) Important to note the trend in readings.
(3) CVP cannot be interpreted on its own.

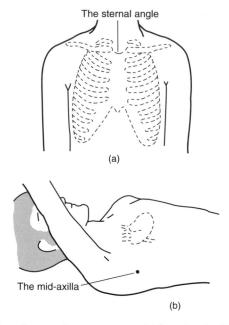

(a)

The sternal angle

The mid-axilla

(b)

Fig. 3.4 Measuring central venous pressure. (a) Sternal angle, (b) mid-axilla.

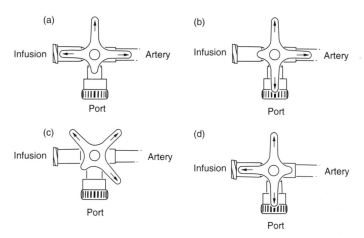

(a) Infusion — Artery — Port

(b) Infusion — Artery — Port

(c) Infusion — Artery — Port

(d) Infusion — Artery — Port

Fig. 3.5 Three-way tap (a) closed to port, (b) turned to artery and port, (c) turned diagonally to close off infusion, artery and port, (d) turned to infusion and port.

Table 3.4 Possible causes for raised and low CVP.

Raised CVP indicates a high blood volume but also.	Lower CVP indicates low blood volume but also.
• Right ventricular failure • Cardiac tamponade • Pulmonary hypertension • Tricuspid valve incompetence • Infusions are in progress during measurements • Catheter tip becoming obstructed or displaced • User error	• Ascites is present (causing raised intra-abdominal pressure). • Vasodilation of peripheral veins is increased. • Vasodilating drugs administered. • Intra-thoracic pressure is raised. • Septicaemia is present. • Sympathetic nervous system dysfunction.

(Manley 1991)

Scenario

Mr Bloggs is a 60-year-old man who is going to require a non-tunnelled central venous catheter prior to going to theatre. He has never been in hospital before and is very anxious.

What can you do to help alleviate his anxiety and what will your role be during the insertion procedure?

Providing an explanation of the procedure that Mr Bloggs will have and why it is necessary will help, as well as showing him an example of the catheter itself, and where, on his body, it may be inserted, e.g. jugular. Explain that he will be lying flat and his head will be tilted, and check that he is able to tolerate this position. Also, go through the Valsalva manoeuvre with him so he understands the importance of it. During the insertion, you will help to position him and perform the Valsalva manoeuvre, as well as being there to reassure him.

CONCLUSION

Non-tunnelled catheters provide an excellent device for those who require immediate central venous access for multiple therapies. However, the benefits must always be weighed up against the risk of the many hazards that can occur, both on insertion and once in situ.

REFERENCES

Baranowski, L. (1993) Central venous access devices – current technologies, uses and management strategies. *Journal of Intravenous Nursing*, **16** (3), 167–194.

Brighton, D. (2004) Observations. In: Dougherty, L. & Lister, L. (eds) *The Royal Marsden Hospital Manual of Clinical Nursing Procedures*, 6th edn. Blackwell Publishing, Oxford.

Crnich, C.J. & Maki, D.G. (2002) The promise of novel technology for the prevention of intravascular device-related bloodstream infections; part 2. Long-term devices, healthcare epidemiology. *Clinical Infectious Diseases*, **34** (10), 1362–1368.

Department of Health (2001) Guidelines for preventing infections associated with the insertion and maintenance of central venous catheters. *Journal of Hospital Infection*, **47** (supplement), S47–S67.

Dougherty, L. (2004) Vascular access devices. In: Dougherty, L. & Lister, S. (eds) *Manual of Clinical Nursing Procedures*, 6th edn. Blackwell Science, Oxford.

Egan Sansivero, G. (1998) Venous anatomy and physiology. Considerations for vascular access device placement and function, *Journal of Intravenous Nursing*, **21** (supplement 5), S107–S114.

Evans Orr, M. (1993) Issues in management of peripheral central venous catheters. *Nursing Clinics of North America*, **28** (4), 911–918.

Gourley, D.A. (1996) Central venous cannulation. *British Journal of Nursing*, **5** (11), 8–15.

Hatchett, R. (2000) Central venous pressure measurement. *Nursing Times*, **96** (15), 49–50.

Henderson, N. (1997) Central venous lines. *Nursing Standard*, **11** (42), 49–54.

Higgins, D. (2004) CVP monitoring. *Nursing Times*, **100** (43), 32–33.

Maki, D.G. (2005) Renowned expert Dennis Maki addresses catheter related infections. *Infection Control Today*, **9** (1). www.infectioncontroltoday.com

Manley, K. (1991) Central venous pressure. *Surgical Nurse*, **4** (5), 10–13.

McPhee, A. (1999) *Handbook of Infusion Therapy.* Springhouse Corporation, Pennsylvania.

Nursing Standard (1999) Quick reference. Guide 6. Central venous lines. *Nursing Standard*, **13** (42), tear-out supplement.

Ostrow, L.S. (1981) Air embolism and central venous lines. *American Journal of Nursing*, (November), 2036–2038.

Scales, K. (1999) Vascular access in the acute care setting. In: Dougherty, L. & Lamb, J. (eds) *Intravenous Therapy in Nursing Practice.* Churchill Livingstone, Edinburgh.

Seldinger, S.I. (1953) Catheter replacement of the needle in percutaneous angiography: a new technique. *Acta Radiologica*, **39**, 368–375.

Seneff, M.G. (1987a) Central venous catheterisation: a comprehensive review; part 1. *Journal of Intensive Care Medicine*, (2), 163–175.

Seneff, M.G. (1987b) Central venous catheterisation: a comprehensive review; part 2. *Journal of Intensive Care Medicine*, (2), 218–232.

Weinstein, S.M. (2001) *Plumer's Principles and Practice of Infusion Therapy.* 7th edn. Lippincott Williams & Wilkins, Philadelphia.

Woodrow, P. (1992) Monitoring central venous pressure. *Nursing Standard*, **6** (33), 25–30.

4 | Skin-tunnelled catheters

The original tunnelled silastic right atrial catheter was developed in the early 1970s by Broviac for home parenteral nutrition (PN). This catheter was fitted with a Dacron® cuff and tunnelled under the patient's skin, from a venous cutdown site to the patient's mid-chest. The Broviac catheter was then modified by Dr Hickman to produce a larger lumen for the administration of blood and blood products, and frequent blood sampling required by bone marrow transplant patients. Despite further modifications, the material and insertion technique remain virtually unchanged (Freedman & Bosserman 1993).

LEARNING OBJECTIVES
By the end of this chapter the reader will be able to:

(1) Define a skin-tunnelled catheter.
(2) List the advantages and disadvantages.
(3) Discuss immediate and follow-up care of the patient.
(4) Describe the removal process.

DEFINITION
A skin-tunnelled catheter is one where the insertion site into the skin is usually on the chest wall, between the nipple and the clavicle, and the catheter is then advanced via a subcutaneous tunnel and inserted along a large central vein until its tip lies in the vena cava or right atrium (see Fig. 4.1a,b) (Royer 2001; Galloway & Bodenham 2004).

TYPES
The most common material used for a skin-tunnelled catheter is silicone. The flexibility and low thrombogenicity make this the preferred material (Davidson & Al-Mufti 1997). The

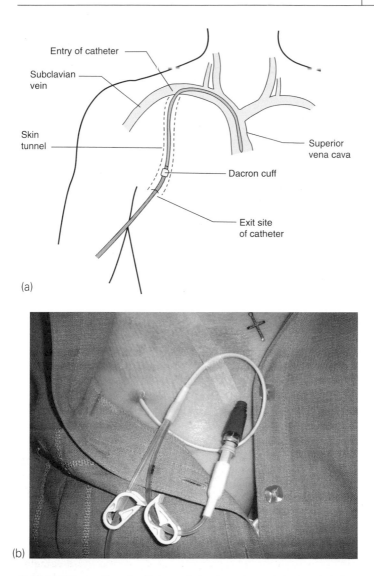

Fig. 4.1 (a) The position of a skin-tunnelled catheter inserted via the subclavian vein. (b) Double lumen skin-tunnelled catheter in situ in a patient.

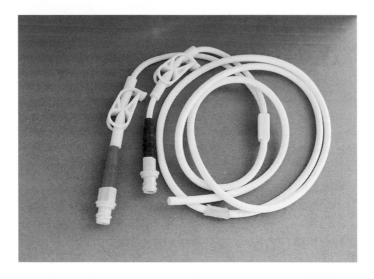

Fig. 4.2 Skin-tunnelled catheter.

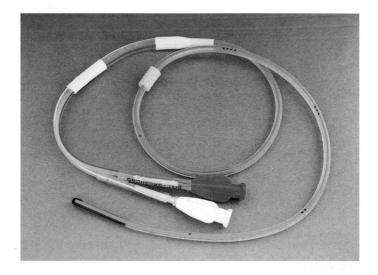

Fig. 4.3 Groshong® valve catheter (Bard).

catheters are available with a single, double or triple lumen (see Fig. 4.2) and can be open-ended or valved (see Fig. 4.3). They are available in a variety of lengths, ranging from 40–90 cm, and open-ended catheters can then be cut to suit the size of the patient. They are available from 5–9 Fr. The inner diameter can be from 0.7–1.6 mm, with a priming volume of 0.3–2.5 ml.

INDICATION FOR USE
These catheters are mainly used for long-term venous access (for months or years) and have been successfully used for:

- parenteral nutrition;
- chemotherapy;
- antibiotics;
- blood and blood products.

ADVANTAGES
The main advantage is their ability to remain in situ for months or years, providing patients with chronic illnesses with reliable venous access. They are also associated with a lower infection rate than a non-tunnelled catheter.

DISADVANTAGES
The main disadvantages are the risk of thrombosis and implications related to body image.

INSERTION

Percutaneous versus surgical technique
Central venous access may be gained either percutaneously (using a needle and guidewire) or via open surgical or cutdown technique. Percutaneous subclavian puncture carries the risk of inadvertent injury to adjacent structures by the needle tip (pneumo/haemothorax or arterial injury), although incidence of complications in experienced units can be kept low. Nightingale et al. (1997) found that the more experienced operators had fewer complications inserting catheters (rates for pneumothorax were 1.8% and for arterial puncture 2.8%). Out of 949 skin-tunnelled catheter insertions, complications necessitating removal were not predicted by age, site of insertion or

malignancy, chemotherapy regimen, platelet or fibrinogen counts, insertion complications or cuff distance from exit site. However, catheters with the tip in the SVC were more at risk of removal than those in the right atrium (2.57 times greater risk). Overall, the complication rate leading to removal was 18.6%: the main causes were infection, thrombosis, migration and pain.

Surgical cutdown avoids the risk of injury to intra-thoracic structures and remains in use, despite longer operating time, and is used in small children (Davidson & Al-Mufti 1997).

INSERTION

Central venous catheterisation is usually accomplished by a percutaneous approach using a Seldinger technique into the subclavian or internal jugular vein. Most tunnelled catheters are inserted using local anaesthetic and conscious sedation. The most common sedation is midazalam (see Chapter 1). It should also be performed under image intensification, which is safer and has greater benefits than the blind landmark technique, particularly in reducing the risk of catheter malposition, as the placement of the wire and catheter is visualised and therefore can be corrected at the time of insertion (Boland et al. 2003). Once the patient is sedated and placed in the Trendelenberg position, the skin is cleaned and then anaesthetised. A relatively large volume of 15–30 ml of 1 or 2% lidocaine is used to distend the tissue planes (Stacey et al. 1991). The addition of adrenaline may help to minimise capillary bleeding and limit local anaesthetic absorption (Pocock 2004). The local anaesthetic is injected at the proposed site of entry into the subclavian or jugular vein and the exit site of the fourth and fifth intercostal spaces between the nipple and sternum.

Once the anaesthesic has taken effect, a small incision is made with a scalpel over the intended venepuncture site. The insertion site should be 1–2 finger breadths below the clavicle, just lateral to where the first rib curves away posteriorly (middle third of clavicle) (Stacey et al. 1991). Insertion too close to the clavicle results in damage to the split sheath introducer and difficulty in threading the catheter. An approach which is too medial may result in a sharp angulation and kinking of the introducer sheath under the clavicle. It will also predispose to pinching between the clavicle and first rib, resulting in pinch off syndrome and possible catheter fracture (Stacey et al. 1991; Galloway & Bodenham 2004).

A needle is then attached to a syringe and inserted via the incision into the vein. Once the vein has been accessed the syringe is disconnected and a J-wire is threaded through the needle. An indication that the wire has been correctly placed is when ectopic beats are seen on ECG and there may be vibration of the wire with each heartbeat. The needle is then removed. The type of catheter will dictate if the tunnel is formed before or after the dilator is advanced along the vein.

An incision is made at the proposed exit site. A tunnelling rod or large trocar is used to form a tunnel under the skin from the exit site to the venpuncture site. Tunnel length and the position of the cuff within the tunnel may vary. Adequate tunnel length and proper location of the cuff are important to avoid displacement of the catheter. The Dacron® cuff elicits a fibrin response, securing the catheter in the subcutaneous tunnel, acting as a mechanical barrier and by increasing anatomical distance from the exit site into the vein, making it more difficult for micro-organisms to reach venous circulation. The subcutaneous tunnel should be about 15 cm in length and the cuff positioned close to the skin exit site (to facilitate catheter removal under local anaesthetic at a later date) and the exit site placed away from any inframammary folds (Davidson & Al-Mufti 1997).

A peel-away sheath introducer and dilator is threaded over the guidewire and advanced into the vein. The guidewire and dilator is removed and the catheter is advanced through the sheath, whilst splitting the sheath. Once the catheter is completely advanced into the vein, the introducer is removed and the catheter should be checked to ensure that blood aspirates easily and there are no problems flushing the catheter. A small skin suture is inserted at the venepuncture site and covered with a small occlusive dressing. At the exit site, a suture is inserted into the skin on either side of the catheter and these sutures are then tied around the catheter to keep it secure whilst fibrous tissue grows around the cuff (Goodman 2000). A dressing is applied.

IMMEDIATE CARE

Once the catheter has been inserted, the dressing over the exit site should be checked for any bleeding. A chest X-ray is usually performed a few hours after insertion to check for pneumothoraces, as well as tip location. The catheter should not be used until the X-ray has been checked, the tip location verified and it has all been documented in the patient's medical and nursing notes.

FOLLOW-UP CARE

The top suture is usually covered with a plaster and the suture is removed after seven days. The padded dressing over the exit site should be changed within the first 24 hours. Thereafter, a transparent dressing is required to cover the exit site until the sutures are removed. This should be changed once a week until the sutures are removed (usually within 2–3 weeks, once a fibroblastic response to the Dacron® has occurred and the catheter is secure). Once the sutures have been removed it is not necessary for a patient to use a dressing. However, some patients prefer to have a gauze dressing over the site to prevent the catheter catching on clothing. If the patient chooses to use a dressing it should be changed every day. Patients should be encouraged to shower every day, and if not then to clean around the exit site with cooled, boiled water and pat dry.

REMOVAL

Prior to removing a skin-tunnelled catheter, the patient should discontinue taking their anticoagulant, such as warfarin, if it was prescribed to prevent thrombosis, usually three days prior to removal. However, if they are on warfarin or any other anticoagulants for a specific reason, e.g. previous thrombosis, they should then be changed to another anticoagulant, such as Fragmin, until the catheter is removed. This can be done if the catheter is to be removed electively, but if the patient needs urgent removal of the catheter, for example in the case of an infection, then vitamin K may be administered prior to removal. These decisions are made based on blood results taken just prior to removal. These include a full blood count to check platelet count and International Normalised Ratio (INR) to check clotting.

There are a range of parameters that need to be checked prior to removal and these may depend on the patient diagnosis and reason for removal, for example with cancer patients the normal range may be a haemoglobin over 10; white blood count over 3 and platelets over 100. The INR should be 1.3 or below (Dougherty 2004). Once the blood results have been deemed acceptable the removal procedure can begin. Patients should have the procedure explained to them and, if required, they may request some sedation such as lorazepam, to help relieve any anxiety. It is very rare for a tunnelled catheter to be removed under a general anaesthetic. There are two main methods for removal of a tunnelled catheter:

(1) traction;
(2) surgical incision and removal.

Traction
This method is carried out by the practitioner applying traction to the end of the catheter and gently pulling to ease the catheter out of the tunnel. This may require a lot of traction and can be uncomfortable for the patient. The greatest risk with this method is that the catheter can snap during traction and then a surgical incision may be required to remove the catheter or, depending on where the break occurs, may necessitate removal by an interventional radiologist. The other problem with this method is that the cuff is often left behind and this can then become a nidus for infection (Drewett 2000; Galloway & Bodenham 2003; Dougherty 2004).

Surgical incision
This method is less hazardous than using traction, but may also be uncomfortable for the patient, and because it requires an incision it will leave a scar. The position of the cuff needs to be identified and in thin patients this may be easily palpable through the skin when the cuff is pulled, as this produces skin tethering, indicating the position of the cuff (Galloway & Bodenham 2003). Alternatively, if the distance of the cuff from

the bifurcation is known then the cuff can be located by using a tape measure (Dougherty 2004). The patient lies flat and local anaesthetic is injected around the cuff. A small incision is then made directly over the cuff and, using forceps, blunt dissection is performed to prise the tissue fibres away from the cuff (Galloway & Bodenham 2004). The catheter is then cut and pulled out. Pressure is applied to the site of insertion into the vessel and also over the incision. Once bleeding has ceased, 2–3 sutures are placed to pull the skin incision together (Galloway & Bodenham 2003). This is then covered with an occlusive dressing, which is left in place for 24 hours (Drewitt 2000). The sutures can be removed after seven days. The patient should remain flat and be observed for a minimum of 30 minutes post-procedure (Galloway & Bodenham 2003).

Scenario

Mr James is a 27-year-old man who has had a fractured femur and requires antibiotics. He has had a skin-tunnelled catheter inserted and is now going home.

What information would you need to communicate to the district nurses who will be caring for him at home?

An initial contact with the district nurse should be made and then written information sent home with the patient, along with all the required equipment for managing the catheter, such as dressings, heparinised saline, etc. The information should cover the types of dressings required, frequency of change, when the sutures should be removed and indications of any complications that may arise and who they should contact if they do occur.

CONCLUSION

Skin-tunnelled catheters have provided a safe and effective central venous access device for many years. Their design has aided in the reduction of infections and they provide long-term venous access for patients requiring a variety of therapies.

REFERENCES

Boland, A., Haycox, A., Bagust, A. & Fitzsimmons, L. (2003) A randomised controlled trial to evaluate the clinical and cost effectiveness of Hickman line insertions in adult cancer patients by nurses. *Health Technology Assessment*, **7** (36).

Davidson, T. & Al-Mufti, R. (1997) Hickman central venous catheters in cancer patients. *Cancer Topics*, **10** (8), 10–14.

Dougherty, L. (2004) Vascular access devices. In: Dougherty, L. & Lister, S. (eds) *Manual of Clinical Nursing Procedures*, 6th edn. Blackwell Science, Oxford.

Drewett, S. (2000) Central venous catheter removal: procedures and rationale. *British Journal of Nursing*, **9** (22), 2304–2315.

Freedman, S.E. & Bosserman, G. (1993) Tunnelled catheters: technologic advances and nursing care issues. *Nursing Clinics of North America*, **28** (4), 851–857.

Galloway, S. & Bodenham, A. (2003) Safe removal of long-term cuffed Hickman-type catheters. *Hospital Medicine*, **64** (1), 20–23.

Galloway, S. & Bodenham, A. (2004) Long-term central venous access. *British Journal of Anaesthesia*, **92**, 722–734.

Goodman, M. (2000) Chemotherapy: principles of administration. In: Henke Yarbro, C. (ed.) *Cancer Nursing*, pp. 385–443. Jones & Bartlett, Massachusetts.

Nightingale, C.E., Norman, A., Cunningham, D., Young, J., Webb, A. & Filshie, J. (1997) A prospective analysis of 949 long-term central venous access catheters for ambulatory chemotherapy in patients with gastrointestinal malignancy. *European Journal of Cancer*, **33** (3), 398–403.

Pocock, M. (2004) The nurses' roles in meeting the vascular access needs of the haematology patient, presented at Intravenous Therapy Within the Cancer Context (9 July, Royal Marsden Hospital national intravenous therapy study day). Royal Marsden Hospital, London.

Royer, T. (2001) A case for posterior, anterior and lateral chest X-rays being performed following each PICC placement. *Journal of Vascular Access Devices*, **6** (4), 9–11.

Stacey, R.G.W., Filshie, J. & Skewes, D. (1991) Percutaneous insertion of Hickman-type catheters. *British Journal of Hospital Medicine*, **46**, 396–398.

5 | Implanted ports

Ports were introduced in the early 1980s for intermittent use in oncology patients, to provide the solution to previous vascular access device problems. Ports are now more versatile and are selected for many more applications (Baranowski 1993). As the port is implanted it can offer patients 'hidden' venous access, but still requires the insertion of a needle.

LEARNING OBJECTIVES
By the end of this chapter the reader will be able to:

(1) Define an implanted port.
(2) Identify the types of ports available and their uses.
(3) List the advantages and disadvantages.
(4) Discuss the types of access needles.
(5) Discuss the implications for the patient.

DEFINITION
An implanted port is a totally implanted venous assess system, comprised of a portal body and a catheter (see Fig. 5.1). The port is a hollow housing of stainless steel/titanium or plastic that contains a compressed latex septum. The portal chamber is connected via a small tube to a polyurethane or silicone catheter that is inserted into a blood vessel. It can remain in place, be functional for many years and is a safe and well tolerated device (Schwarz et al. 1997; Brown et al. 1997; Goodman 2000).

TYPES OF PORTS AND ACCESS NEEDLES
There are a variety of ports: venous, arterial, intraperitoneal and epidural. Venous ports (see Fig. 5.2) are available in both adult and paediatric sizes. The range of ports include standard ports, low profile ports (these are useful for long-term

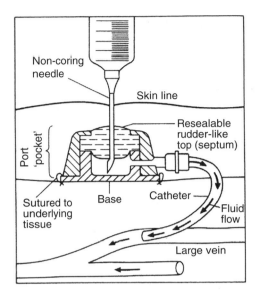

Fig. 5.1 Cross-section of an implantable port accessed with a non-coring needle.

access, especially when a patient is concerned about the port being obvious showing through the skin), top or side entry ports (useful when patients require access for long infusions, as the side entry port allows a more secure placement of the needle, with a reduced risk of dislodgement) (McPhee 1999).

The portal body is made of titanium or plastic (stainless steel ports were discontinued with the advent of MRI scanning) and these do not cause any problem during MRI (McPhee 1999; Weinstein 2001). The port septum is made of silicone, as is the catheter. Ports are available with pre-attached or attachable catheters (which is usually connected to the portal body by means of a locking ring) in single and double designs. A double port has two distinct portal chambers to allow simultaneous administration of separate solutions. Peripheral ports combine the properties of a PICC and a port. They are half the size of a

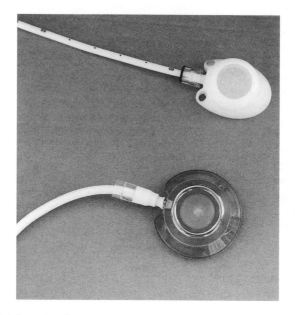

Fig. 5.2 Examples of venous ports.

standard port and allow patients to experience the advantages of a peripherally placed device (less invasive) with the portal body being located in the upper arm (Goodman 2000). Catheter lumen tips can be open-ended or valved.

Needles

The needles used to access a port are specially designed to prevent damage to the portal septum. They have a flattened or offset bevel and are called non-coring or Huber needles (Fig. 5.3; McPhee 1999; Weinstein 2001; Gabriel 2004). They are available in gauge sizes from 19–22g, and lengths ranging from 15–25mm (see Fig. 5.4a). They can be integral to an extension set, or can be configured as a winged infusion set (see Fig. 5.4b).

The following should be considered when selecting a needle (McPhee 1999):

(1) depth of port (may need a longer needle if port is very deep);
(2) location of port;
(3) type of therapy required (a large gauge may be required for viscous fluids, e.g. blood);
(4) speed of infusion;
(5) length of time port needs to be accessed;
(6) who is accessing the port.

USES

Ports can be used for the same reasons as any other CVAD and are viewed as a long-term access device, which can be managed successfully for both home and hospital therapy. They are easy to maintain and have few complications (Dougherty 2004).

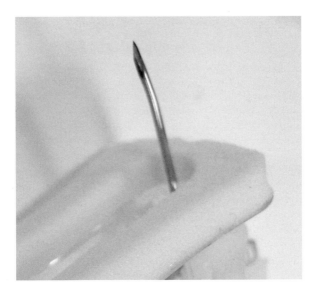

Fig. 5.3 Gripper Plus® Safety Needle, showing the non-coring bevel, courtesy of Smiths Medical.

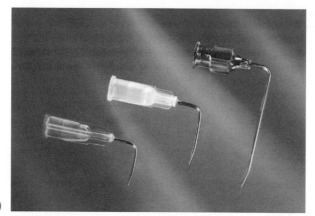

(a)

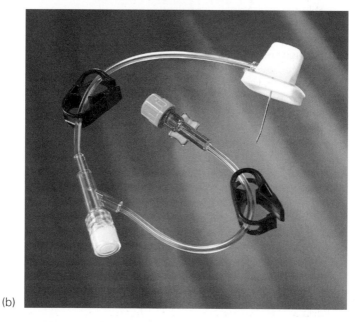

(b)

Fig. 5.4 (a) 90° Huber needles of different gauge sizes, (b) Gripper® Needle with a winged infusion set, both images courtesy of Smiths Medical.

ADVANTAGES

The main advantage ports have over any of the other devices is that they are implanted and are therefore not external to the body. This is an advantage for a number of reasons:

(1) Patient's body image: the literature supports the impact on body image when comparing ports with external catheters. In one study, patients showed less problems relating to body image when they had a port in situ, when compared with those who had a tunnelled catheter. However, those with ports that were very superficial and were easily observed through the skin, demonstrated similar patterns of body image problems to those with tunnelled catheters (Mirro et al. 1989). Therefore, the location of the port can be vital.
(2) It requires minimal manipulation: ports only require flushing once a month when not in use, making them more suitable for intermittent therapies.
(3) This reduction in manipulation may, in turn, result in reduced risk of infection. Studies showed that when comparing ports (in solid tumour patients) with tunnelled catheters (in haematology patients), patients with ports acquired fewer infections (Richard Alexander 1994). Initially, ports are expensive in terms of cost implantation, but least expensive for routine care and maintenance (Schwarz et al. 1996; Brown et al. 1997; Goodman 2000).

DISADVANTAGES

One disadvantage of ports is that most practitioners choose to insert them under general anaesthetic (GA) so a patient must be fit enough to undergo a GA. The scarring on insertion and removal is more extensive than with any other device. Ports cannot be repaired if they become damaged. They are associated with a risk of needlestick injury to staff, as a needle is left in situ, although manufacturers are now developing safety needles, where a needle shield is activated once the needle is withdrawn from the port.

Ports are also associated with the highest risk of extravasation, when compared with other CVADs (Hallquist Vaile 2003). This, in itself, leads to another disadvantage, in that staff who access ports need to be trained in order to ensure the port is accessed correctly and to reduce the risk of extravasation or infiltration. This means that some patients will have to attend a local centre where trained staff are available. If this is not an option, patients may have to undergo treatments or tests without using the port, due to lack of availability of trained staff, or be prepared to learn to access the ports themselves. All these issues must be discussed with patients prior to port insertion. Finally, this device still requires that the patient has a needle inserted to gain access to the port, and whilst many patients are happy for a local anaesthetic cream to be applied to the port prior to accessing, for some who may be needle phobic, this would not be the ideal device.

Location of a port

The decision of where a port is located on the patient's body is often related to who will be accessing the device. If patients are accessing their own port then it should be located low on the rib cage for easy access. When patients are not accessing their own ports then the port is usually located on the upper rib cage near the clavicle (Fig. 5.5a). Ports near the sternum provide better needle stability and ease of access. If the patient is to access the port it should be placed on a firm surface, ideally over a rib, to provide support for access and stability, making it easy for the patient to visualise care, but it should not be visible when the patient is clothed. Adequate subcutaneous tissue will prevent erosion through the skin. If the port is placed too deeply or there is excess adipose tissue it can make access difficult. In a thin patient a low profile port should be used, whilst a large port should be used in obese patients or large breasted women. Placement under the arm, in the breast or the soft tissue of the abdomen should be avoided (Goodman 2000).

INSERTION

This is usually carried out under general anaesthetic. Ports are available:

(1) With catheter previously attached to the portal housing; in which case the surgeon trims the distal end off prior to insertion.

(2) With the catheter separate from portal housing; in which case the surgeon trims the proximal end prior to attaching and securing it to the portal body during implantation.

The surgeon makes an incision and the port is placed subcutaneously and sutured into a subcutaneous pocket, usually in the infraclavicular fossa above the pectoralis major fascia. The catheter is then tunnelled. The vessel is selected as for a tunnelled catheter and the catheter threaded until its tip is located in the superior vena cava. If it is placed in the saphenous vein then it is advanced to the inferior vena cava and the port is placed on top of the thigh (Baranowski 1993; McPhee 1999; Weinstein 2001; Dougherty 2004). Peripheral ports allow peripheral insertion. Once the catheter is placed, the portal body is subcutaneously implanted below the antecubital fossa (Camp Sorrell 1992).

The incision is then sutured and dressed. The suture line should not be over the port, but made 3–5 cm from the top of the port, so that the practitioner does not have to insert the access needle through the suture line. It should be accessed prior to leaving the theatre if it is to be used immediately, as the area will be tender and oedematous, causing manipulation to be uncomfortable. Some practitioners prefer to wait 14 days prior to accessing the port, to allow post-operative oedema to resolve and the wound to heal (Goodman 2000).

IMMEDIATE CARE
Once the port has been inserted, the dressing over the sutures/ incision site should be checked for any bleeding. A chest X-ray is usually performed a few hours after insertion to check for pneumothoraces, as well as tip location. The port should not be used until the X-ray has been checked, the tip location verified and all the relevant information has been documented in the patient's medical and nursing notes.

FOLLOW-UP CARE
Once the port is accessed the needle can remain in situ for a period of seven days (Fig. 5.5b). It should then be removed, and if the patient requires ongoing therapy the port can be

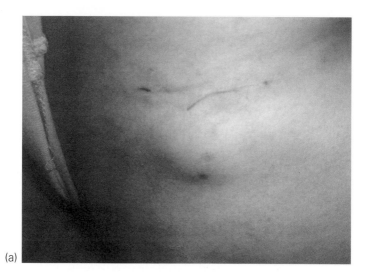

(a)

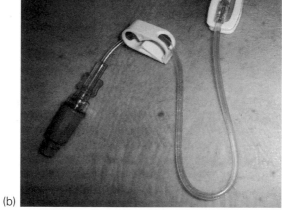

(b)

Fig. 5.5 (a) Implanted port of a patient's chest, (b) implanted port accessed in a patient.

reaccessed with a new needle. The needle should be supported to prevent any trauma to the skin, and also to prevent dislodgement. Selecting the correct length and type of needle can help to reduce this (McPhee 1999; Weinstein 2001; Dougherty 2004). A transparent dressing should then be placed over the port and the needle, which can be changed at needle change or as necessary. If the port is not accessed, once the sutures have dissolved or been removed, no further care is required by staff or patient. The port will be flushed once a month with a heparinised saline solution: 100 iu per ml, to a total of 5 ml (McPhee 1999; Weinstein 2001; Dougherty 2004). It is stipulated by the manufacturers of ports that only 10 ml syringes or larger should be used for any drug administration and this includes the flushing solution. This is to prevent pressure being generated from smaller syringes, which could cause disconnection between the portal body and the catheter or catheter damage (Conn 1993; McPhee 1999; Weinstein 2001; Dougherty 2004).

REMOVAL
This is usually carried out under general anaesthetic. The port is removed by making an incision into the dense fibrous sac which forms round the port in the longer term. There are usually four small anchoring sutures attaching the port to the deeper tissues. These are cut and the port is then removed (Galloway & Bodenham 2004). Skin sutures are inserted and these are usually removed at seven days.

Scenario

John Pringle is a 36-year-old man with AIDS, and he had a port inserted so that he could administer his antifungal treatments at home. These need to be given twice a day and he has not had any problems. He initially lost weight, but now has regained some and he reports to the hospital that during his last infusion, he could not feel the needle hit the backplate of the port and now the port looks red and inflamed.

What could have happened and what actions should be taken?

It may be that due to his weight gain, the needles he was using are now no longer long enough to reach the port and remain in situ safely. The needle may have dislodged during his last infusion, and some of the drug may have leaked into the tissues. The extravasation will need to be referred to the medical team, and once it has healed, the correct length needles should be supplied and these should be reviewed on a regular basis to ensure they remain suitable.

CONCLUSION

Ports provide patients with a totally implanted central venous access device. This means that for those who may be required to have a CVAD for the rest of their lives, they can continue their normal activities, with less aspects of care for such a device. Along with the body image benefits, ports are usually a successful and well-liked CVAD.

References

Baranowski, L. (1993) Central venous access devices – current technologies, uses and management strategies. *Journal of Intravenous Nursing*, **16** (3), 167–194.

Brown, D.F., Muirhead, M.J., Travis, P.M., Vire, S.R., Weller, J. & Hauer Jensen, M. (1997) Mode of chemotherapy does not affect complications with an implantable venous access device. *Cancer*, (80), 966–972.

Camp Sorrell, D. (1992) Implantable ports: everything you always wanted to know. *Journal of Intravenous Nursing*, **15** (5), 262–273.

Camp Sorrell, D. (1994) Magnetic resonance imaging and the implantable port. *Oncology Nursing Forum*, **17** (2), 197–199.

Conn, C. (1993) The importance of syringe size when using an implanted vascular access device. *Journal of Vascular Access Networks*, **3** (1), 11–18.

Dougherty, L. (2004) Vascular access devices. In: Dougherty, L. & Lister, S. (eds) *Manual of Clinical Nursing Procedures*, 6th edn. Blackwell Science, Oxford.

Gabriel, J. (1999) Chapter 11 Long-term central venous access. In: Dougherty, L. & Lamb, J. (eds) *Intravenous Therapy in Nursing Practice*, pp. 301–332. Churchill Livingstone, Edinburgh.

Galloway, S. & Bodenham, A. (2004) Long-term central venous access. *British Journal of Anaesthesia*, **92**, 722–734.

Goodman, M. (2000) Chemotherapy: principles of administration. In: Henke Yarbro, C. (ed.) *Cancer Nursing*, pp. 385–443. Jones & Bartlett, Massachusetts.

Hallquist Viale, P. (2003) Complications associated with implantable vascular access devices in the patient with cancer. *Journal of Intravenous Nursing*, **26** (2), 97–102.

McPhee, A. (1999) *Handbook of Infusion Therapy*. Springhouse Corporation, Pennsylvania.

Mirro, J., Rao, B.N., Stokes, D.C. & Austin, B.A. (1989) A prospective study of Hickman/Broviac catheters and implantable ports in paediatric oncology patients. *Journal of Clinical Oncology*, **7**, 214–222.

Richard Alexander, H. (1994) Clinical performance of long-term venous access devices. In: Richard Alexander, H. (ed.) *Vascular Access in the Cancer Patient: Devices, Insertion Techniques, Maintenance and Prevention and Management of Complications*, pp. 18–36. J.B. Lippincott, Philadelphia.

Schwarz, R.E., Groeger, R.S. & Coit, G. (1997) Subcutaneously implanted central venous access devices in cancer patients. *Cancer*, (79), 1635–1640.

Weinstein, S.M. (2001) *Plumer's Principles and Practice of Infusion Therapy*. 7th edn. Lippincott Williams & Wilkins, Philadelphia.

6 | Management of CVADs

The key principles in the managing of CVADs are the same, whichever device is in situ. These are: the prevention of infection (by use of aseptic techniques, cleaning solutions and dressings), maintaining patency and preventing damage.

LEARNING OBJECTIVES
By the end of this chapter the reader will be able to:

(1) Discuss the importance of securing and dressing a CVAD.
(2) Discuss the rationale for maintaining patency.
(3) List what should be assessed during site inspection and why.
(4) Describe how to take blood samples, and identify potential problems.

SECUREMENT AND DRESSING

Securement
Ports are implanted and tunnelled catheters usually have a cuff to secure the device, so the main types requiring ongoing securement during the time they are in situ are PICCs and non-tunnelled CVCs.

Securing a central venous access device is vital in preventing complications (see Table 6.1). Securing the device prevents the catheter moving and becoming displaced. Movement at the insertion site can cause mechanical irritation and lead to phlebitis. Excessive movement can result in a pyogenic granuloma, especially at the insertion site of a PICC. Movement of the catheter in and out can also act like a piston and may encourage micro-organisms on the skin to be pulled in via the venepuncture site and either track along the outside of the catheter

Table 6.1 Complications of poor securement.

- Catheter migration
- Phlebitis
- Infection
- Damaged catheters

(Gabriel 2001)

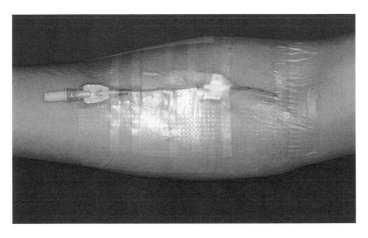

Fig. 6.1 PICC secured with Statlock™ and transparent dressing. Image courtesy of Bard Ltd.

(tunnelled catheter) or enter the venous circulation, leading to infection and possible septicaemia.

There are a number of skin securement devices. Sterile strips such as Steristrips™ are available in different widths and can help to maintain securement of a PICC (see Fig. 6.1). Most non-tunnelled central venous catheters are designed with suture holes, usually found in the wings, to allow for suturing. Skin-tunnelled catheters are fixed to the skin by suturing through the skin and then tying the sutures around the catheter. These remain in situ until there has been adequate granulation along the tunnel tract. These sutures are usually removed 2–3 weeks after insertion, as they are no longer required. The disadvantages of suturing are that it can be uncomfortable, can result in scarring and may contribute to increasing infection (Gabriel 2001). It is now recommended that sutures are not used to secure CVC because of the increased risk of infection (Maki 2002; RCN 2003).

Securement devices, which are made specifically for the purpose of securing CVCs, and now available, such as Statlock™ (see Fig. 2.3). Stacey (2000) found that they prevented migration and found no documented incidence of infection during their use. Gabriel (2001) reported that patients found them comfortable. They have been shown to be effective in maintaining the security of the catheters (Yamamoto et al. 2002; Schears 2005), reducing local complications, such as phlebitis, and reducing the risk of bloodstream infections (Crnich & Maki 2002). They also do not appear to result in any scar tissue formation (Gabriel 2001). Moureau & Iannucci (2003) found that using an adhesive pad with an integrated retainer designed to hold a catheter in place, offered more security than tape. They reviewed a number of studies and found that when comparing tape and securing devices, such as Statlock™, in both peripheral devices and CVADs (such as PICCs), results showed that catheter dislodgement was greatly reduced (in 67%), complications were reduced (50%) as well as unscheduled restarts (78%). Catheter dwell times were also increased (53%). Securement of needles into ports is also important to reduce the risk of extravasation, infiltration and needlestick injury, as well as local trauma to skin and portal septum.

Dressings

Once the catheter has been secured then a sterile dressing should be placed over the securement device and the catheter at the insertion site.

The purpose of a dressing is to:

(1) Provide protection of the catheter insertion site from external contamination.
(2) Secure the CVC to prevent dislodgement and trauma.
(3) Discourage bacterial proliferation near the insertion site.

The ideal dressing for any intravenous device should provide all the properties listed in Table 6.2.

When choosing a dressing Woods et al. (2000) highlighted the properties that should be considered:

- Which dressing maintains the integrity of the vascular site?
- Which factors influence the dressing integrity?
- What is the nurse's preference for ease of application and removal of dressing?
- Which dressing is cost effective related to product and nursing time?
- What impact would the dressing have on CVC infection rates?

There has been much debate related to intravenous dressings in the last 20 years. Lau (1996) carried out a review of dressings, mainly gauze and transparent dressings. She noted that research results on catheter related sepsis were influenced by the following:

- adherence to, and frequency of, aseptic technique;
- skin preparation;
- site of insertion;
- duration of catheterisation;
- age;
- sex;
- amount of moisture at insertion site;
- type of dressing material.

Engervall et al. (1995) found that clinical and bacteriological data indicated that changing polyurethane CVC dressings twice

Table 6.2 Ideal dressing properties.

- Be sterile
- Provide an effective barrier to bacteria
- Allow the catheter to be securely fixed
- Easy to apply and remove
- Be comfortable for the patient

(RCN 1992; Finley 2004)

a week was superior to once week in haematology patients. Little (1998) compared Opsite IV 3000™ with a standard dressing, i.e. dry dressing, and looked at the bacteriological data, as well as staff experiences with the dressings. She found no statistically significant difference in the incidence of catheter-related infections but more staff preferred the Opsite IV 3000™. The main disadvantages were that it was problematic with clammy skin, which necessitated its removal due to the lack of adhesion in these patients, and some staff highlighted having difficulty in removing the dressing.

Reynolds et al. (1997) carried out a study comparing Tegaderm™ and Opsite IV 3000™. Patients were randomly assigned each dressing, and the insertion site and amount of fluid under the dressing was assessed at each dressing change. These were performed every two days, and on removal of the catheter in CCU patients. There was no statistically significant difference between the two dressings in accumulation of fluid, skin microbial colonisation, local infection or systemic infection when the dressing was changed every two days. However, more work needs to be carried out on the differences over 5–7 days (Treston Aurend et al. 1997).

It is believed that cutaneous microflora at the insertion site account for the majority of catheter related infections (Maki & Ringer 1987). They compared a transparent dressing (TD) with tape and gauze (T & G) and highly permeable transparent dressing (HPTD). Benefits of the HPTD included: easy visualisation of insertion site; increased adherence capacity and prevention of moisture accumulation. They found that in the TD versus HPTD group there was a significant difference, showing a lower catheter related infection rate with the HPTD and that there was up to a 25% reduction in catheter related infections. Jones (2004) found that highly permeable transparent dressings were well tolerated by patients and were easy to apply and remove. The RCN (2003) recommended the use of a transparent moisture permeable dressing with all CVADs, stating that it should be changed within the first 24 hours following insertion and then weekly thereafter.

Gillies et al. (2003) carried out a systematic review and concluded that there was no evidence of any difference in the incidence of infectious complications between any of the dressing types compared in their review. Jones (2004) concluded her review of dressings with the recommendation that in choosing an intravenous dressing, staff should be aware of the advantages and disadvantages of the current dressings on the market in order to make an informed choice.

SITE INSPECTION

Whenever a dressing is changed the site should be inspected for any signs of infection, infiltration, extravasation or phlebitis. Complaints of soreness, unexpected pyrexia and damaged, soiled or wet dressings are reasons for immediate inspection and renewal of the dressing (Dougherty 2004). See Table 6.3 for a list of the features that should be assessed (Egan Sansivero & Barton Burke 2002).

MAINTAINING PATENCY

Patency is defined as:

(1) ability to infuse through a catheter;
(2) ability to aspirate blood from a catheter.

Table 6.3 List of features which should be assessed at dressing change.

Skin and tract
- Skin condition
- Presence and character of any drainage
- Skin colour, temperature and sensation
- Integrity of Huber needle (where appropriate)
- Integrity of dressing
- Presence of oedema, collateral vessel
- Device

Integrity
- Presence of clamp
- Tubing, cap and extension set security
- External length
- Presence of blood return

Securing devices
- Security of skin securing device/sutures

(Egan Sansivero & Barton Burke 2002)

Catheter occlusions are said to occur when either of these criteria cannot be met (Krzywda 1999). Maintaining patency is a role for the nurse and the patient who may be caring for their own CVAD. It is based on the correct solution in the correct volume and given at the correct intervals. Success is also related to the method or technique used to maintain patency.

Solutions

The two common solutions for maintaining patency are:

(1) 0.9% sodium chloride;
(2) heparinsed saline.

The literature is clear on the subject of the solution to use with peripheral cannulae. However, there has not been as much work carried out to look at maintaining patency in CVADs. Certainly, there are few comparative studies using the two solutions. Kelly et al. (1992) found that flushing once a week with heparinised saline was adequate to maintain patency in tunnelled catheters in haematology patients. The DoH (2001) and NICE (2003) both support the use of a heparinised saline solution, although neither of them states the concentration of heparin. The common concentration is 10 iu per ml, with a total of 50 iu given within a four-hour period. The disadvantages of heparin are well documented and include iatrogenic haemorrhage, allergy, and cost (Goode 1991; Dougherty 2004).

The solution of 0.9% sodium chloride has always been advocated for flushing prior to use of a catheter to check patency. It is used between the administration of drugs to ensure that no mixing of drugs occurs, and therefore reduces the risk of incompatibility reactions, and flushed at the end of drug administration to ensure all of the drug has been administered. However, whether it should be used primarily for maintaining patency is unclear. Manufacturers of valved catheters, such as the Groshong® valved catheter recommend that 0.9% sodium chloride is adequate to maintain patency (Weinstein 2001; RCN 2003). Nevertheless, it appears that heparinised saline is still the recommended solution for use with open-ended catheters (RCN 2003; NICE 2003). A stronger concentration is recommended for use with implantable ports, where most manufacturers recommend 100 iu per ml to a total of 500 iu (Dougherty 2004).

Volume
The internal volume of a catheter will differ depending on the design of the catheter and its length. Open-ended catheters can be cut, so even the internal volume listed by the manufacturers will alter, depending on the final length of catheter inserted into the patient. This does not help the practitioner when deciding on the volume of flush to be used for maintaining patency. There are lists of total internal volume for certain types of catheters, which can provide some guidance, but on average a skin-tunnelled catheter in an adult has an internal volume of 1.5–2 ml with a PICC having 0.5–1 ml.

The standard volume of pre-prepared heparinised saline is 5 ml (50 iu). However, the volume of 0.9% sodium chloride varies. It is usually recommended that about 5 ml is used to check patency, and in between drugs 2–5 ml, but this may be dependent on the drugs being given and the capacity for interactions. At the end of drug administration 5 ml is standard, and then 5–10 ml to maintain patency. This is not harmful to a patient unless the catheter is being used repeatedly and there are issues related to the size of the patient, e.g. a child, any restrictions on fluids or problems related to sodium intake (RCN 2003; Dougherty 2004; Finley 2004).

Frequency of flushing
Flushing with 0.9% sodium chloride is performed as described above, when using the catheter to administer drugs. However, the frequency of flushing when the device is not in use is a controversial issue. One view is that the more times the device is manipulated the more risk there is of contaminating it and increasing the risk of infection. This risk must be weighed against the need to ensure the device remains patent. Most centres now flush CVCs once a week (RCN 2003; Dougherty 2004). However, in implanted ports it is recommended that flushing need only occur once a month (McPhee 1999; RCN 2003).

Method of flushing
There are two main methods for maintaining patency that are highlighted by the literature:

(1) Turbulent or pulsatile flush (produces turbulence and reduces the potential for material to stick inside or at tip of catheter).
(2) Positive pressure (prevents retrograde movement of blood back into the catheter).

Goodwin & Carlson (1993) described the pulsatile flush method as being the most effective method to clear the catheter of any blood or drugs that may adhere to the internal lumen of the catheter. It can be achieved by administering the flushing solution in short bursts or pulses (e.g. 0.5–1 ml at a time). Instead of laminar flow, which only results in flushing of the central portion of the catheter, this method promotes turbulence within the lumen, which is more effective.

Positive pressure
Positive pressure is a technique used to prevent the reflux of blood into the distal tip of the catheter (Moureau 1999). If a catheter is flushed, as the syringe is disconnected from the distal end then a small volume of fluid shifts back into the syringe, which in turn means that blood may have refluxed into the tip. This can then result in an occlusion. Positive pressure is achieved by maintaining pressure on the plunger with a thumb, as the syringe is disconnected, thus creating a positive pressure within the catheter (Dougherty 2004). This is effective, but if not performed correctly can still result in occlusion. For this reason, manufacturers have developed a needle-free positive displacement injection cap, which is attached to the end of the lumen providing the benefits of a closed needle-free system and creating the positive pressure required to maintain patency (see Figs 6.2a,b). Berger (2000) found that using positive pressure devices resulted in a significant decrease in the incidence of catheter occlusion, which in turn significantly reduced the cost of patient care. Lenhart (2001) also found the use of these caps reduced CVAD occlusions.

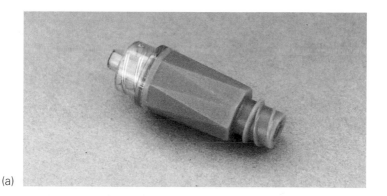

(a)

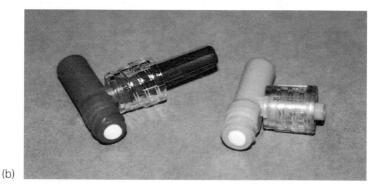

(b)

Fig. 6.2 (a) Posiflow positive pressure injection cap. (b) CLC 2000 positive pressure injection cap.

TAKING BLOOD SAMPLES

There is a view that a central venous access device should not be used for blood sampling as this can increase the risk of infection. Theoretically this is possible, particularly if the catheter is not flushed in the correct manner. Blood withdrawn through the catheter can adhere to the internal lumen and if not flushed completely can provide a great nidus for bacterial growth and may also result in occlusion (Ernst & Ernst 2001). However, in a large number of patients with CVADs one of the main benefits is the ability to use it for obtaining blood samples. Blood sampling should be performed using syringes or a vacuum system. The vacuum system does provide less risk of blood contamination, the correct volume and removes the necessity for decanting blood. However, sometimes the vacuum can cause collapse of the catheter, particularly if the catheter is silicone, and some manufacturers do not recommend its use on PICCs or in implanted ports.

It is usual to use the proximal lumen of a multi-lumen catheter, and where these catheters have different sized lumens, to use the largest lumen for blood sampling. Sometimes a lumen will be labelled for blood sampling only, so that there is no risk of contamination of the sample (Weinstein 2001; Dougherty 2004). If an infusion is in progress on a single lumen catheter then it may be necessary to discontinue the infusion and then obtain the blood sample, but this will be dependent on what is being administered and the patient's condition. If a lumen is not free in a multi-lumen catheter then the lumen containing the infusion that will have the least risk of contamination of the sample and be the safest to discontinue should be used. In devices where the lumen exits are staggered along the length of the catheter it is suitable to take a blood sample whilst other infusions are in progress. However, it may be necessary to stop all infusions whilst the sample is being obtained.

A procedure for blood sampling is outlined in Table 6.4.

Due to the risk of small clots being present within the lumen of the catheter, one view is that prior to flushing the catheter, a specified volume of blood (usually 5 ml) should be withdrawn and discarded. However, the literature to support this is not conclusive. Anderson Johnson et al. (1987) state that there is evidence that micro-clots have been found when withdrawing blood from a lumen, but the clinical relevance of flushing these clots into the patient is not clear. For this reason, and the problems that can result if blood cannot be obtained on withdrawal (risk of potential occlusion, increased patient anxiety), the risks outweigh the benefits, and the view is that it is unnecessary to withdraw blood prior to flushing. This is supported by the RCN Standards for Infusion Therapy (2003). However, this should

Table 6.4 Procedure for blood sampling from a CVAD.

(1) Explain the procedure to the patient and check request forms to ascertain sample bottles required and to check patient's identity.
(2) Gather all necessary equipment.
(3) Wash hands with bactericidal soap and water or bactericidal alcohol handrub.
(4) Apply non-sterile gloves (for protection of practitioner).
(5) If using a needle-free injection cap, clean the end with a chlorhexidine alcohol solution and allow to dry.
If using an injectable cap then remove the cap and clean the lumen end as above.
(6) If using a vacuum system:
 (a) attach the adaptor to the shell;
 (b) push vacuumed bottle onto adaptor and discard first sample bottle to prevent contamination of samples;
 (c) take samples as required (see Fig. 6.3).
(7) If using a syringe:
 (a) attach syringe and withdraw 10 ml of blood and discard;
 (b) attach clean syringe and take appropriate volume of blood for samples required;
 (c) decant blood into the bottles.
(8) Following sampling, flush the lumen with a minimum of 10 ml of 0.9% sodium chloride, using a pulsatile flush to ensure adequate clearance of blood.
(9) Apply new cap if appropriate.
(10) Flush the catheter with the appropriate flushing solution, e.g. heparinised saline, using pulsatile flush and ending with positive pressure.
(11) Label bottles and place into appropriate containers and send to the laboratory.
(12) If blood cannot be obtained consider the following:
 (a) patient's position;
 (b) probability of fibrin sheath or precipitation;
 (c) possible tip malposition.

not be confused with the withdrawal of blood prior to blood sampling.

There are a number of methods of blood sampling to ensure that the blood sample is not contaminated with 0.9% sodium chloride and heparin:

(1) discard method;
(2) mixing method;
(3) reinfusion method.

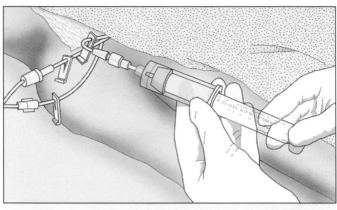

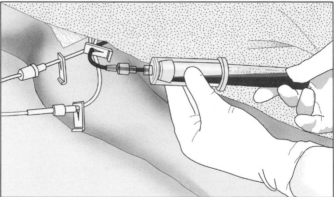

Fig. 6.3 Obtaining a blood sample using a vacuum system. Redrawn from McPhee, A. (1999) *Handbook of Infusion Therapy* with permission of Lippincott Williams & Wilkins.

Discard method

This is when a small volume of blood is withdrawn from the catheter and discarded prior to taking the requested blood samples. The problem with this method is the volume taken, especially if the patient has a low circulating volume, such as in children, or in hypovolemic or anaemic patients. It is also debatable how much blood should be taken as a discard sample, which is usually cited as 3–6 ml. The discard samples can be obtained using a vacuum bottle or a syringe: the syringe exposes the practitioner to a risk of blood contamination, but it may be that the bottle is more expensive if more than one is to be discarded (Cosca et al. 1998; Holmes 1998).

Mixing method
This involves attaching a syringe to the lumen of the catheter and withdrawing and reinfusing the sample 4–6 times to 'mix' the contents of the lumen with the blood, to clear the catheter of any heparin or intravenous fluids and finally, to achieve a clean sample. This reduces the risk of infection and blood loss. There is, however, a risk of haemolysis of the sample and risk of contamination when decanting (Cosca et al. 1998; Holmes 1998).

Reinfusion method
This consists of taking a sample of blood in a syringe, usually about 6 ml, to clear the catheter of any heparin or intravenous fluids. That syringe is then capped off with a sterile cap and set aside, the required blood samples are taken and then the first sample is reinfused. This helps to prevent loss of blood and is useful in paediatrics. However, there are issues over the time the blood is left, the risk of contamination and the possibility of clot formation (Frey 2002).

Keller (1994) found that the majority of bone marrow transplant units use the discard method, and that volumes removed and discarded ranged from 0.5–10 ml. Their concerns were the risk of infection and blood loss, and the accuracy of laboratory results. Pinto (1994) compared coagulation values drawn from heparinised CVC and peripheral veins and found that accurate coagulation values cannot be obtained from a CVC, even after a volume of six times the dead space volume was withdrawn. Hinds et al. (2002) also found that neither a 6, 9 nor 12 ml discard, from a heparinised CVAD, was sufficient to yield a clinically trustworthy coagulation study. Holmes (1998) compared the discard and mixing methods and found no difference between the methods. A reduction in blood loss, exposure to staff, potential specimen contamination and erroneous reporting were benefits of the mixing method.

Table 6.5 General principles related to CVC blood sampling methods.

Discard	• Always flush prior to obtaining specimen and use discard when obtaining drug levels. • Consider removal of at least three times the catheter volume to clear the catheter of infusate. • If removing discard with syringe, use a new syringe to obtain sample. • Label one as discard prior to drawing sample to avoid confusion.
Reinfusion	• Method may introduce a clot into the system, although whether clots present in the catheter and reinfusion represent a significant risk is unclear.
Mixing	• May be accurate for tests other than coagulation and drug levels. • Drug levels and coagulation.

Literature does not support drawing blood for coagulation through a heparinised CVAD, particularly if monitoring anticoagulant therapy.

Frey (2002) presented a review of all the methods and studies and recommended the following general principles to the method used (see Table 6.5).

It must be noted that when blood culture samples are required, no matter what method is chosen, the first sample of blood should be used.

The literature does not support the use of silicone central venous catheters for sampling drug levels if the drug is being given via the same catheter. In general, if a double lumen catheter is used, it is recommended that the larger lumen is used for blood withdrawal and infusions should be stopped prior to blood sampling. However, it is important that the nurse should ensure that the device is flushed off to prevent occlusion whilst the infusion is switched off.

On occasions, a catheter may not bleed. This may be due to a number of reasons:

(1) *Position*: a catheter can become positional and this is often dependent on tip location. The tip may be resting on the wall of the vein or it may be that the tip is too far into right

atrium. Encouraging the patient to take a deep breath or tilting their head down often helps. It may also be necessary for them to move their arm into a different position. However, if this is the case then the pinch off syndrome should be considered (see Chapter 8).

(2) *Fibrin sheath*: fibrin builds up along the length of the catheter within hours of the catheter being inserted. This may not cause any problems initially but a fibrin sleeve at the tip or a fibrin tail may result in problems with blood withdrawal. This is often referred to as a persistent withdrawal occlusion (see Chapter 7). An instillation of a fibrinolytic agent usually resolves this problem. Fibrin sheath is the most common reason for a catheter not bleeding.

(3) *Tip malposition*: this will require further investigation and possible chest X-ray to verify tip location (see Chapter 7).

Scenario

Miss Pear, aged 33, who has lymphoma, has had a skin-tunnelled catheter in situ for five months and is on her last course of chemotherapy. She needs blood samples taken prior to her treatment, but there is no blood return, although the 0.9% sodium chloride flush is injected easily.

What could be the cause of the lack of blood return and what steps should be taken prior to administering any chemotherapy?

This is likely to be a persistent withdrawal occlusion, which may be due to position, fibrin sheath formation or malposition of the tip. The patient should be repositioned and take deep breaths to ascertain if it is positional. If this does not work, it may be necessary to challenge the device with fluid to see if there is any discomfort or swelling which may indicate damage or problems with the location of the tip. Urokinase can be instilled to aid in breaking down any fibrin and, finally, a chest X-ray may be ordered to ascertain tip location.

CONCLUSION

There are certain principles, which should be applied whatever the device: prevent infection, maintain patency and prevent damage. If these principles are followed, then the care and management of CVADs is made relatively easy.

REFERENCES

Anderson Johnson, A., Krasnow, S.H., Boyer, M.W., Racheisen, M.L., Grant, C.E., Gasper, O.R., Hoffman, J.K. & Cohen, M.H. (1987) Hickman catheter clots: a common occurrence despite daily heparin flushing. *Cancer Treatment Reports*, **71** (6), 651–653.

Berger, L. (2000) The effects of positive pressure devices on catheter occlusions. *Journal of Vascular Access Devices*, **5** (4), 31–33.

Cosca, P.A., Smith, S., Chatfield, S., Meleason, A., Muir, C.A., Neratzis, S., Petrofsly, M. & Williams, S. (1998) Reinfusion of discard blood from venous access devices. *Oncology Nursing Forum*, **25** (6), 73–76.

Crnich, C.J. & Maki, D.G. (2002) The promise of novel technology for the prevention of intravascular device-related bloodstream infections; part 2. Long-term devices, healthcare epidemiology. *Clinical Infectious Diseases*, **34** (10), 1362–1368.

Department of Health (2001) Guidelines for preventing infections associated with the insertion and maintenance of central venous catheters. *Journal of Hospital Infection*, **47** (supplement), S47–S67.

Dougherty, L. (2004) Vascular access devices. In: Dougherty, L. & Lister, S. (eds) *Manual of Clinical Nursing Procedures*, 6th edn. Blackwell Science, Oxford.

Egan Sansivero, G. & Barton Burke, M. (2002) Chemotherapy administration: general principles for vascular access. In: Barton Burke, M., Wilkes, G. & Ingwerson, K. (eds) *Cancer: a Nursing Process Approach*, pp. 645–670. Jones & Bartlett, Massachusetts.

Engervall, P., Ringertz, S., Hagman, E., Skogman, K. & Bjorkholm, M. (1995) Change of central venous catheter dressings twice a week is superior to once a week in patients with haematological malignancies. *Journal of Hospital Infection*, (29), 275–286.

Ernst, D. & Ernst, C. (2001) *Phlebotomy for Nurses and Nursing Personnel*. Health Star Press, Indiana.

Finley, T. (2004) *Intravenous Therapy*. Blackwell Publishing, Oxford.

Frey, A.M. (2002) Drawing labs from venous access devices. National Association of Venous Access Networks 15th annual conference, Virginia.

Gabriel, J. (2001) PICC securement: minimise potential complications. *Nursing Standard*, **15** (43), 42–44.

Gillies, D., O'Riordan, E., Carr, D., O'Brien, I., Frost, J. & Gunning, R. (2003) Central venous catheter dressings: a systemic review. *Journal of Advanced Nursing*, **44** (6), 623–632.

Goode, C.J. (1991) A meta-analysis of the effects of heparin flush and saline flush – quality and cost implications. *Nursing Research*, **40** (6), 324–330.

Goodwin, M. & Carlson, I. (1993) The peripherally inserted central catheter: a retrospective look at three years insertions. *Journal of Intravenous Nursing*, **16** (2), 92–103.

Hinds, P.S., Quargnenti, A., Gattuso, J., Srivasta, D.C., Tong, X., Penn, L., West, N., Cathey, P., Hawkins, D., Williams, J., Starr, M. & Had, D. (2002) Comparing the results of anticoagulation tests on blood drawn by venepuncture and through heparinised tunnelled venous devices in paediatric patients with cancer. *Oncology Nursing Forum*, **29** (3), 477.

Holmes, K.R. (1998) Comparison of push-pull versus discard method from central venous catheters for blood testing. *Journal of Intravenous Nursing*, **21** (5), 282–285.

Jones, A. (2004) Dressings for the management of catheter sites – a review. *Journal of Association of Vascular Access*, **9** (1), 1–8.

Keller, C.A. (1994) Method of drawing blood samples through central venous catheters in paediatric patients undergoing bone marrow transplant. *Oncology Nursing Forum*, **21** (5), 879–884.

Kelly, C., Dumenko, L., McGregor, S.E. & McHutchion, M.E. (1992) A change in flushing protocol of CVC. *Oncology Nursing Forum*, **19** (4), 599–605.

Krzywda, E.D. (1999) Predisposing factors, prevention and management of central venous catheter occlusions. *Journal of Intravenous Nursing*, **22** (supplement), S11–S17.

Lau, C.E. (1996) Transparent and gauze dressings and their effect on infection rates of central venous catheters: a review of past and current literature. *Journal of Intravenous Nursing*, **19**, 240–245.

Lenhart, C. (2001) Prevention versus treatment of vascular access device occlusions. *Journal of Vascular Access Devices*, **5** (4), 34–35.

Little, K. & Palmer, D. (1998) Central line exit sites: which dressing? *Nursing Standard*, **12** (48), 42–44.

Maki, D.G. (2002) The promise of novel technology for prevention of intravascular device related bloodstream infections. National Association of Vascular Access Networks conference presentation (Sept.). San Diego.

Maki, D.G. & Ringer, M. (1987) Evaluation of dressing regimes for prevention of infection with peripheral intravenous catheters. *Journal of American Medical Association*, **258** (17), 2396–2403.

McPhee, A. (1999) *Handbook of Infusion Therapy.* Springhouse Corporation, Pennsylvania.

Moureau, N. (1999) Practising prevention with implanted ports. *Journal of Vascular Access Devices*, **4** (3), 30–35.

Moureau, N. & Iannucci, A.L. (2003) Catheter securement: trends in performance and complications associated with the use of either traditional methods or adhesive anchor device. *Journal of Vascular Access Devices*, (Spring), 29–33.

National Institute for Clinical Excellence (NICE) (2003) *Infection Control Prevention of healthcare associated infection in primary and community care*, Clinical Guidelines 2. Department of Health, London.

Pinto, K.M. (1994) Accuracy of coagulation values obtained from a heparinised central venous catheter. *Oncology Nursing Forum*, **21** (3), 573–575.

Reynolds, M.G., Tebbs, S.E. & Elliott, T.S.J. (1997) Do dressings with increased permeability reduce the incidence of central venous catheter related sepsis? *Intensive and Critical Care Nursing*, (13), 26–29.

Royal College of Nursing and Infection Control Nurses Association (1992) *Intravenous Line Dressings – Principles of Infection Control.* Smith & Nephew Medical Ltd, Hull.

Royal College of Nursing Intravenous Therapy Forum (2003) *Standards for Infusion Therapy.* Royal College of Nursing, London.

Schears, G.J. (2005) The benefits of a catheter securement device on reducing patient complications. *Managing Hospital Infection*, **5** (2), 14–20.

Stacey, R.G.W. (2000) Percutaneous insertion of Hickman-type catheters. *British Journal of Hospital Medicine*, **46**, 96–98.

Treston-Aurend, J., Olmsted, R.N., Allen-Bridson, K. & Craig, C.P. (1997) Impact of dressing materials on central venous catheter infection rates. *Journal of Intravenous Nursing*, **20** (4), 201–206.

Weinstein, S.M. (2001) *Plumer's Principles and Practice of Infusion Therapy.* 7th edn. Lippincott Williams & Wilkins, Philadelphia.

Woods, S.S., Nass, J. & Deisch, P. (2000) Selection and implementation of transparent dressings for central vascular access devices. *Nursing Clinics of North America*, **35** (2), 385–393.

Yamamoto, A.J., Solomon, J.A., Soulen, M.C., Tang, J., Parkinson, K., Lin, R. & Schears, G.J. (2002) Sutureless securement devices reduce the complications of peripherally inserted central catheters. *Journal of Vascular and Interventional Radiology*, **13** (1), 77–81.

Hazards of insertion

7

The insertion of a central venous catheter is not without its hazards and is not a procedure to be undertaken lightly (see Table 7.1). The benefits and risks should be considred prior to insertion and any risk factors reduced by correcting any deficits, to ensure that the patient is in an optimal condition to undergo the procedure.

LEARNING OBJECTIVES
By the end of this chapter the reader will be able to:

(1) List the hazards that can occur during insertion.
(2) Identify the signs and symptoms of the most common complications that may occur.
(3) Discuss the prevention and management for each complication.

HAZARDS OF CENTRAL VENOUS CATHETERISATION

PNEUMOTHORAX
Pneumothorax means presence of air in the pleura (Scales 1999; Perdue 2001; Weinstein 2001; Dougherty 2004). It can occur for a number of reasons, but is the commonest complication with central venous catheterisation. It results from the puncture of the pleura during the insertion of a central venous catheter. It is usually related to the vein used for cannulation and is more common with the subclavian approach, due to its anatomical proximity to the lung. It is characterised by shortness of breath and sudden onset of chest pain but the patient may be asymptomatic and it may only be discovered on the chest X-ray performed following the procedure. Other symptoms include tachycardia, persistent cough and diaphoresis (Perdue 2001).

Table 7.1 Complications that can occur during insertion of a CVAD and once in situ.

On insertion	Once in situ
• Pneumothorax	• Infection
• Haemothorax	• Thrombosis
• Haemorrhage	• Malposition
• Haematoma	• Occlusion
• Air embolism	• Catheter damage
• Brachial nerve plexus	• Extravasation
• Malposition	
• Catheter embolism	

Prevention

The more skilled the practitioner is, the less likely it is that a pneumothorax will occur (Nightingale et al. 1997). However, there are now guidelines published with respect to new technology that can greatly help to reduce the risk of pneumothorax (NICE 2003). The use of two-dimensional ultrasound imaging prior to, during and after insertion can guide the practitioner. It enables him to visualise the desired vein, and check vessel patency and position, especially in relation to other organs and vessels. The procedure can then be performed under ultrasound guidance, enabling the visualisation of the vessel and the needle once it enters the vein, ensuring that the risk of a through puncture (and subsequent puncture of the lung) is reduced.

Management

If symptoms are noted during insertion the practitioner may stop the procedure. The patient's colour, respirations and pulse should be monitored and oxygen should be administered. In the case of a small pneumothorax, the patient may feel slightly breathless, but no intervention is required and the pneumothorax will heal spontaneously. However, if it is a large pneumothorax then the patient will require the insertion of a chest drain (Perdue 2001) (see Table 7.2).

Table 7.2 Signs and symptoms of a pneumothorax and nursing care.

Signs and symptoms	Nursing care
Dyspnoea, shortness of breath	Monitor respiratory rate and report if increasing significantly. Provision of oxygen, sit patient upright when procedure allows and if air embolism not suspected.
Oxygen desaturation of arterial blood	Monitor oxygen saturation via peripheral probe throughout. Administer oxygen. Assist in arterial blood sampling and be ready to assist with insertion of chest drain to re-inflate lung.
Wheezing	Sit upright, if procedure allows. Administer nebulisers as prescribed.
Dry cough	Encourage patients to take shallow breathes to avoid coughing.
Pain on inspiration/expiration	Administer analgesia as prescribed. Assist with comfortable positioning.
Asymmetrical chest movement	Assist with positioning of patient to allow medical staff to listen to breath sounds. Be prepared to assist in insertion of chest drain.
Tracheal deviation	Support patients during investigation and treatment.

(Reproduced with permission from Drewett, S. (2000) Complications of CVC nursing care. *British Journal of Nursing*, **9**(8); 468.)

HAEMOTHORAX

A haemothorax, in this context, is when blood enters the pleural cavity as a result of trauma or transection of a vein during insertion of a central venous catheter. The patient may experience a sudden onset of chest pain with mild to severe dyspnoea during catheter insertion. However, the patient may be asymptomatic as symptoms depend on the amount of blood released into the cavity. Delayed symptoms include tachycardia, hypotension, skin colour changes and haemoptysis.

Prevention

Prevention is similar to that for a pneumothorax: a skilled practitioner, correct positioning of the patient and good education to ensure compliance during the procedure.

Management

If symptoms are noted during catheter insertion the practitioner should remove the catheter and apply pressure to the site. Vital signs should be monitored and symptoms treated. If symptoms occur after the catheter has been inserted, the medical team should be informed immediately (Perdue 2001).

HAEMORRHAGE/ARTERIAL PUNCTURE

A haemorrhage or arterial puncture is uncontrolled bleeding, in this context, as a result of damage to the vein and/or artery during or following insertion of a CVC. It is not usually a serious problem unless the carotid artery is punctured (Perdue 2001).

Prevention

The use of ultrasound can help to reduce the risk of arterial puncture and the artery can be visualised during insertion. It is important to ensure that the patient is not compromised by: having a high International Normalised Ratio (INR), receiving anticoagulant therapy or having a low platelet count. These should all be corrected by administration of platelets, administration of vitamin K, stopping medication a few days prior to insertion, or changing the patient from warfarin to subcutaneous low molecular weight heparin, e.g. Fragmin.

Management

If symptoms are noted at the time of insertion and the artery can be located, then pressure should be applied for at least five minutes (longer if the patient has a bleeding disorder). Pressure is not always possible as the ability to apply pressure depends on the location of the artery (Perdue 2001). If symptoms are not recognised immediately then the patient may develop a mediastinal haematoma, which can then lead to tracheal compression and respiratory distress (Perdue 2001).

HAEMATOMA

A haematoma is uncontrolled bleeding at the venepuncture site, creating a hard painful lump. This may occur during insertion of the introducer needle prior to PICC or CVC insertion (Lamb 1999; Perdue 2001; Dougherty 2004).

Prevention

A haematoma can be avoided by knowledge of patients who may be more susceptible to haematoma formation, e.g. patients with low platelet counts, or who are on anticoagulants. Following insertion, any at-risk patient should be placed back into the supine position to prevent an increased risk of haematoma.

Management

The needle should be removed and pressure applied to the area. Where appropriate, the extremity can be elevated. The site should be monitored. Ice packs can be applied (Perdue 2001; Witt 2004). The patient should be informed of what has occurred and educated to report any changes in sensation, which could occur if bleeding has occurred deeper into the tissues and is causing pressure on the nerves.

AIR EMBOLISM

Venous air embolism is the entry of air into the venous system as a consequence of trauma or iatrogenic complications, especially CVC catheterisation or pressurised intravenous infusion systems (Ostrow 1981). It can also occur following various surgical procedures and on removal of a central venous catheter. During insertion, large introducers are used (a 14g needle allows air at 200 ml into the vein), and this enables air to be drawn into the central circulation in large amounts, very rapidly. This puts the patient at greatest risk at this time, especially when the dilator is disconnected at the hub in order to advance the catheter into the vein. It is also more likely to occur if the patient is hypovolemic, when patients are vulnerable, such as critically ill patients, and in those gasping for air.

Air drawn into the central system results in right ventricular dysfunction and pulmonary injury (Conrad 2002). Small amounts of air do not produce symptoms because air is removed from the circulation. Large boluses of air (3–8 ml/kg) can cause acute right ventricular outflow obstruction and result in cardiogenic shock and circulatory arrest. If air is drawn in at a rate of 70–105 ml of air per second it is usually fatal, and at 20 ml a patient will experience symptoms (Mennim et al. 1992), so the small bubbles found in intravenous tubing are not usually a problem.

Incidence

The true incidence is unknown. A sub-clinical air embolism in hospitalised patients is possibly quite common. Frequency of clinically recognised air embolism following CVC is less than 2% (Conrad 2002). Symptomatic air embolism, following CVC, has a mortality rate as high as 30%.

Symptoms

These tend to develop immediately following embolisation; the severity of the symptoms is related to the degree of air entry and include (Drewett 2000a):

- dyspnoea;
- chest pain;
- tachycardia;
- hypotension;
- confusion;
- anxiety;
- lowered levels of consciousness;
- neurological deficits;
- circulatory shock or sudden death.

Prevention

- Proper positioning of the patient during insertion and removal. This should be with the head tilted lower than the feet in a position known as a Trendelenberg, which helps to engorge the veins, and if air does enter it prevents it from travelling to the heart. The patient performing the Valsalva manoeuvre can also reduce the volume of air that might enter.

- Whilst it would be ideal to have the patients rehydrated prior to CVC insertion, often the procedure is performed during emergency situations when the patient is bleeding and collapsed and, in effect, requires the catheter in order to receive the fluid and/or blood. However, wherever possible ensure that the patient is not hypovolemic as this can also generate an increased 'sucking' force.

- Use a closed CVC system and maintain vigilance during manipulation, as it can occur during accidental disconnection and dislodgement. It is therefore recommended that only Luer Lok connections should be used, to reduce the risk of disconnection.

- Air embolism can also occur during removal, when air can enter the catheter tract between the catheter and sealing of the tract. The degree of risk is related to the length of time in situ, as the longer it has been in the vein, the longer the tract takes to seal (Ostrow 1981), although it can occur after a CVC has been in as little as three days. It may be delayed for 30 minutes or more. The initial dressing after removal must be occlusive, and using Valsalva during disconnection can also increase intra-thoracic pressure as well as increasing main pressure within the central vein (Ostrow 1981; Scales 1999) (see Table 7.3).

Management

Staff should resist the temptation to sit a breathless patient upright, in the case of a suspected air embolism the management is to lie them in the left lateral (recovery position) with the head lower than the feet (Trendelenberg). This manoeuvre helps to trap air in the apex of the ventricle, prevents ejection into the pulmonary arterial system and maintains right ventricular output (see Fig. 7.1a,b) (Ostrow 1981). Administer 100% oxygen and intubate if there are signs of respiratory distress. If an air embolism is suspected during CVC procedure, the procedure should be terminated. The patient should then be placed in the Trendelenberg and left lateral position.

BRACHIAL NERVE PLEXUS INJURY

The brachial nerve plexus is a network of lower cervical and upper dorsal spinal nerves, which supply the arm, forearm and

Table 7.3 Steps for reducing risk of air on catheter removal.

Action	Rationale
Ensure the patient is not dehydrated	A low CVP will allow air to be aspirated into the systemic circulation more easily.
Position patient in the Trendelenberg position (10–30° head down tilt).	This position elevates the venous pressure above that of atmospheric pressure, thus reducing the risk of air being aspirated.
Remove when patient performs the Valsalva maneoeuvre.	The pressures involved within the central venous circulation relate directly to the pressures involved with respiration. On expiration the intra-thoracic and intravenous pressures are greater than the atmospheric pressure, making it less likely that air would enter the venous system. On inspiration it is the opposite, and air can be sucked in through an opening into the venous system.
Apply gentle pressure to occlude exit site of catheter for five minutes unless clotting deranged.	Pressure will prevent both blood loss and air entry. Compression can disrupt a blood clot within the venous system, or if over the carotid artery it can cause neurological or cardiopulmonary complication.
Apply airtight dressing for at least 24 hours and encourage patient to lie down for a minimum of 30 minutes.	When the patient first sits up or takes a deep breath the CVP will be increased to above air pressure. The dressing will prevent air being sucked in while the tract seals.

(Reproduced with permission from Drewett, S. (2000) CVC removal procedures and rationale. *British Journal of Nursing*, **9**(22), 2306.

hand (Perdue 2001). Due to their anatomical position they may be injured during catheter insertion. Patients may experience tingling sensations in the fingers, or pain shooting down the arm, or paralysis.

Management
The doctor should be informed and administer analgesia as required. Physiotherapy may be helpful, but it does not always resolve the injury (Perdue 2001).

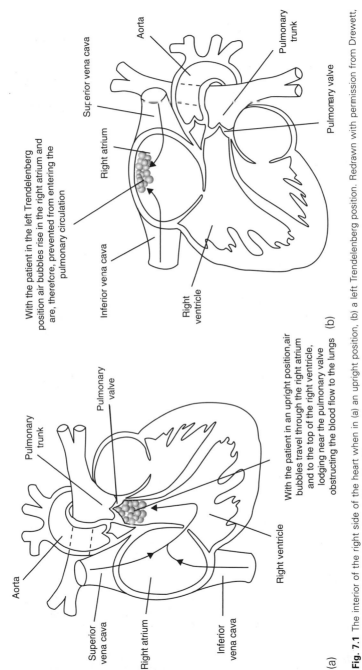

With the patient in the left Trendelenberg position air bubbles rise in the right atrium and are, therefore, prevented from entering the pulmonary circulation

Aorta

Pulmonary trunk

Pulmonary valve

Superior vena cava

Right atrium

Inferior vena cava

Right ventricle

(b)

With the patient in an upright position, air bubbles travel through the right atrium and to the top of the right ventricle, lodging near the pulmonary valve obstructing the blood flow to the lungs

Pulmonary trunk

Pulmonary valve

Aorta

Superior vena cava

Right atrium

Inferior vena cava

Right ventricle

(a)

Fig. 7.1 The interior of the right side of the heart when in (a) an upright position, (b) a left Trendelenberg position. Redrawn with permission from Drewett, S. (2000b). *British Journal of Nursing*, **9** (8), 466–478.

CATHETER MALPOSITION

A catheter malposition is when the catheter tip is not in, or is no longer in, the correct position, and will depend on where the tip was placed initially, or where the tip placement was desired, e.g. in the SVC. A catheter may become malpositioned during insertion or at any time whilst in situ.

Incidence

Malposition can occur in 21–55% of insertions (Ingle 1995). Placement via the basilic vein results in a greater chance of malposition into the internal jugular vein. It occurs during insertion, guidewire exchange, or can occur spontaneously. Newer catheter materials predispose to greater frequency of looping, coiling or knotting in the vein.

During insertion

The catheter may have been inadvertently inserted into large tributaries of the SVC, e.g. jugular system, internal mammary, azygous, superior intercostal and pericardiophrenic veins. It may be more common via the left brachiocephalic than the right (as this vein is more oblique, longer and has a larger number of tributaries). However, it may reduce the risk of malposition into the jugular vein. Inadvertent cannulation of small venous tributaries has been associated with pericardial chest pain, mid-thoracic back pain and shoulder pain, each intensified by hypertonic solutions. Omission of the lateral view on CXR may result in failure to detect a malpositioned catheter.

Difficulty advancing the catheter or anatomical deviances may result in the tip ending in the jugular vein, being coiled in the subclavian or axillary vein, going across into the opposite brachiocephalic vein, or being advanced too far into the right atrium or ventricle. It may also be that the catheter has advanced into completely the wrong vein as into the azygous vein. Some clues may indicate wrong placement during insertion, such as the patient complaining of sensory sensations, a 'gurgling' during advancement or during flushing of the catheter (jugular placement), or a 'fluttery' feeling in the chest, or palpitations (catheter in atrium or ventricle). Difficulty advancing or not getting blood return during insertion could indicate coiling.

Once in situ
Catheter migration out of the superior vena cava can occur from days to months following insertion, or can occur spontaneously, although it is unclear why. Possible causes include vigorous upper extremity use, forceful flushing at the catheter, congestive heart failure, catheter foreshortening and changes in intra-thoracic pressure caused by coughing, emesis, or constipation. Malposition may also occur as a result of Twiddler's syndrome. This syndrome is characterised by intentional or unintentional manipulation of a subcutaneous port or catheter, and may lead to the catheter being 'removed' from the vein. The syndrome may be an indication of a patient's anxiety, as they are often unaware of their manipulation (Ingle 1995).

Signs and symptoms

- Can be asymptomatic.
- Partial or complete catheter occlusion.
- Chest/shoulder or back pain, with infusion.
- Reduced infusion rate.
- Signs of extravasation.
- Ipsilateral extremity oedema.
- 'Ear gurgling', described by patients with a catheter malpositioned in the internal jugular vein.
- Backflow of blood into external tubing unrelated to increased intra-thoracic pressure.
- Resistance or discomfort during insertion.
- Kink in guidewire when removed from catheter.

Malposition may be diagnosed due to the catheter becoming longer at the exit site or the cuff showing (in a tunnelled catheter, especially following pulling of catheter), more exposed catheter at the insertion site of a PICC or no blood return. Any of these would lead the practitioner to question tip placement. In order to obtain a definitive diagnosis the catheter must be X-rayed to verify tip location. This may necessitate a lateral as well as the standard PA view on chest X-ray (see Figure 1.8).

Prevention

On insertion of a PICC, check that the head is correctly positioned to prevent jugular placement, and carry out a thorough assessment of the patient for any anatomical issues, history of previous difficulties inserting the catheter, or fractured clavicles. There should also be accurate measurement to prevent placement in RA or ventricle. Once in situ there should be adequate securement of the device, both at the site and also of the extension sets, education of the patient to ensure that it is not pulled and to report early if there are any changes to the length of the external portion of the catheter.

Management

During insertion, if malposition is suspected it can be rectified. Ultrasound of the jugular vein can indicate malposition in the vessel prior to sending the patient for an X-ray. If the wire is left in during PICC insertion or in a polyurethane catheter, the malposition can be rectified, or an over the guidewire exchange can take place. Other techniques for rectifying malposition include:

- Positioning, such as sitting patient upright.
- Rapid flush, during insertion.

Once in situ, some may resolve spontaneously and return to the correct position. Difficult placements can be performed under X-ray, or may require repositioning using fluoroscopy (Ingle 1995). Guidance or use of an interventional radiologist may also correct coiled or malpositioned catheters. If it cannot be corrected then removal may be necessary, and is preferable if therapies include vesicant or hypertonic solutions, or if the patient reports pain.

Scenario

You have just sat Mr Dixon up after removing his central venous catheter, and he has now developed shortness of breath, chest pain and is looking cyanosed. He is tachycardic and hypotensive and is showing signs of confusion.

What could the cause of his symptoms be and what should be done?

He may now be suffering from an air embolism. It is impor tant that he is not sat upright, but placed in the left lateral position with his head lower than his feet (Trendelenberg). This will prevent any air travelling to the lungs. Administer oxygen and call for assistance. Ensure that there is an airtight transparent dressing over the venepuncture site to prevent further air entry. Reassure Mr Dixon as he will be very anxious.

CONCLUSION
Prevention of complications is the key. However, even when all preventative actions are taken, complications can still occur and it is imperative that the nurse can recognise them as early as possible and take the appropriate management action to prevent further injury or the removal of the device.

REFERENCES
Conrad, S.A. (2002) Venous air embolism. *eMedicine Journal*, **3** (4). www.emedicine.com

Dougherty, L. (2004) Vascular access devices. In: Dougherty, L. & Lister, S. (eds) *Manual of Clinical Nursing Procedures*, 6th edn. Blackwell Science, Oxford.

Drewett, S. (2000a) Central venous catheter removal: procedures and rationale. *British Journal of Nursing*, **9** (22), 2304–2315.

Drewett, S. (2000b) Complications of central venous catheters: nursing care. *British Journal of Nursing*, **9** (8), 466–478.

Ingle, R.J. (1995) Rare complications of vascular access devices. *Seminars in Oncology Nursing*, **11** (3), 184–193.

Lamb, J. (1999) Local and systemic complications of intravenous therapy. In: Dougherty, L. & Lamb, J. (eds) *Intravenous Therapy in Nursing Practice*. Churchill Livingstone, Edinburgh.

Mennim, P., Coyle, C.F. & Taylor, J.D. (1992) Venous air embolism associated with removal of central venous catheter. *British Medical Journal*, (305), 171–172.

National Institute for Clinical Excellence (NICE) (2003) *Infection Control Prevention of Healthcare Associated Infection in Primary and Community Care*, Clinical Guidelines 2. Department of Health, London.

Nightingale, C.E., Norman, A., Cunningham, D., Young, J., Webb, A. & Filshie, J. (1997) A prospective analysis of 949 long-term central venous access catheters for ambulatory chemotherapy in patients with gastrointestinal malignancy. *European Journal of Cancer*, **33** (3), 398–403.

Ostrow, L.S. (1981) Air embolism and central venous lines. *American Journal of Nursing*, (November), 2036–2038.

Perdue, M.B. (2001) Intravenous complications. In: Carlson, K., Perdue, M.B. & Hankins, J. (eds) *Infusion Therapy in Clinical Practice*, 2nd edn. W.B. Saunders, Pennsylvania.

Scales, K. (1999) Vascular access in the acute care setting. In: Dougherty, L. & Lamb, J. (eds). *Intravenous Therapy in Nursing Practice*. Churchill Livingstone, Edinburgh.

Weinstein, S.M. (2001) *Plumer's Principles and Practice of Infusion Therapy*, 7th edn. Lippincott Williams & Wilkins, Philadelphia.

Witt, B. (2004) Venepuncture. In: Dougherty, L. & Lister, S. (eds) *The Royal Marsden Hospital Manual of Clinical Nursing Procedures*, 6th edn. Blackwell Publishing, Oxford.

Managing complications

8

More than 15% of patients who undergo central venous catheterisation have complications once the catheter is in situ. These include mechanical complications (5–19%), infectious (2–26%) and thrombotic (2–26%) (McGee & Gould 2003). Nurses have an important role in detecting and treating them promptly to reduce their effects and, wherever possible, to prevent them.

LEARNING OBJECTIVES
By the end of this chapter the reader should be able to:

(1) List the common complications associated with CVADs, once in situ.
(2) Describe the causes of the complications.
(3) List ways of preventing the complications.
(4) Discuss the management of each complication, should they arise.

CATHETER DAMAGE
Catheter damage can occur at different points along the catheter:

(1) The catheter hub.
(2) The catheter near the hub or below a bifurcation.
(3) The catheter, higher up the catheter, or above a bifurcation.
(4) Internal catheter fracture.

The position of the catheter damage will dictate whether the catheter can be repaired or needs to be removed (Dougherty 2004).

Damage at the catheter hub

'Overscrewing' of a cap onto the hub, or applying the cap to the hub, which has been cleaned with alcohol, but not allowed to dry adequately (which effectively 'glues it on', causing difficulty when removing), can both result in cracking of the hub. This can be repaired easily by removing the damaged hub and replacing it, but does require the selection of the correct hub for the correct catheter. However, the ability to repair the hub will depend on the type of catheter, as some have hubs which are integral to the catheter and cannot be repaired (Dougherty 2004).

Damage near the hub or below the bifurcation

This can occur if the wrong types of clamps are used. Silicone is a fragile material, prone to damage; therefore only the clamps provided with the catheter or smooth-bladed forceps should be used. Artery or toothed forceps can cause small breaks in the wall of the catheter. Damage done to this section of the catheter can be repaired by adding a small sleeve to the area of damage and gluing it into place. This should only be considered to be a temporary repair and the catheter should be replaced as early as possible, due to the risk of contamination of the catheter. In some cases, such as PICCs, the catheter can be shortened by cutting off the damaged portion and reapplying a new hub. This type of repair will need to be considered in respect to the tip location, as shortening the catheter will result in a new tip location and a chest X-ray must be performed to verify the exact tip location (Ingle 1995; Dougherty 2004).

Damage higher up the catheter or above the bifurcation

This can occur on insertion and may only be discovered once an infusion is commenced, but it occurs more commonly as a result of 'nicking' the catheter when sutures are removed at the exit site, or if small syringes are used to unblock a catheter and the pressure results in small holes or splits in the catheter. When a skin-tunnelled catheter is damaged the only solution is removal of the catheter. Exchange over a guidewire may be carried out with non-tunnelled catheters or single lumen PICCs.

This is performed by cutting the end off the catheter, threading a guidewire along the catheter to a specified distance, removing the catheter and threading a new catheter, via an introducer, into the vein. This can only be performed if there are no signs of infection and requires the use of special guidewires, dilators and introducers (Dougherty 2004).

Internal catheter fracture

This can result from damage caused during insertion by the practitioner, but more commonly as a result of pinch off syndrome (Ingle 1995; Andris & Krzywda 1997a). Pinch off syndrome occurs when the catheter becomes trapped between the clavicle and the first rib (Fig. 8.1). The rubbing may result in damage occurring over a period of time and finally resulting in fracture of the catheter and catheter embolism.

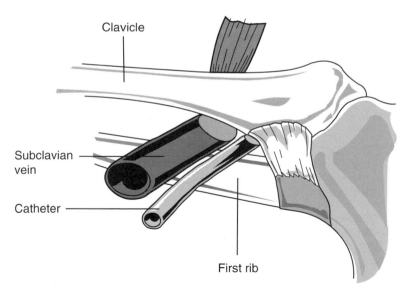

Fig. 8.1 Diagram to illustrate pinch-off syndrome. Redrawn from Macklin, D. & Chernecky, C. (2004) *IV Therapy*. Saunders, St Louis. With permission of Elsevier.

Prevention of damage

Damaged catheters result in removal of a working device, distress and discomfort for the patient, and time delay in treatment, as well as cost. Prevention is the key, and the use of the correct equipment when manipulating the catheter, managing occluded catheters appropriately and taking care when handling the catheter all help to prevent damage (Ingle 1995; Andris & Krzywda 1997a).

Catheter repair

This can only be performed in external catheters. Implanted ports have no external segment to repair and any fracture will require surgical replacement. Currently non-tunnelled catheters have no repair segments commercially available and so the best remedy is to exchange the catheter over a guidewire. Skin-tunnelled catheters and some PICCs can be repaired, and this should be carried out in accordance with the manufacturer's instructions (Reed & Philips 1996).

Catheter fracture and catheter embolism

There are a number of causes of catheter fracture and subsequent embolism:

(1) Separation of the catheter from the port, forceful flushing in the presence of distal obstruction, manufacturing defect, or incorrect locking procedure.
(2) Catheter shear from needles/sutures or surgical instruments during insertion.
(3) On removal using traction or against excessive resistance.
(4) Catheter pinch off syndrome (Drewett 2000).

Pinch off syndrome occurs when a CVC is inserted percutaneously via the subclavian vein and it becomes compressed by the clavicle and the first rib (Andris & Krzywda 1997a; Verhage & van Bommel 1999). It results in:

(1) intermittent mechanical obstruction of the catheter;
(2) complete or partial catheter transection;
(3) possible catheter embolisation into the central venous system (Ingle 1995).

The anatomy of the axillary subclavian vein and costo-clavicular space, the puncture site and approach angle are all critical to its development (Ingle 1995; Andris & Krzywda 1997a). It is only seen in percutenous subclavian placements (see Fig. 8.1). Although PICCs pass this area, they are not at risk of pinch off. Attention to surgical technique during placement can reduce the incidence, and the ideal location for subclavian insertion is lateral to the mid-clavicular line. This syndrome is often unrecognised and under-reported. The reported incidence is listed as between 0.1–1.12%. It is frequently identified by clinicians retrospectively, after associated complications, such as catheter fracture. There is a high index of suspicion in the following situations:

- catheter is positional;
- weak points in catheter 'balloon out' (Ingle 1995; Macklin & Chernecky 2004).

Clinical symptoms consistent with pinch off syndrome include:

- difficulty in aspirating blood (PWO);
- resistance to flushing of infusion: intermittent occlusion relieved by rolling the shoulder or raising the arm on the ipsilateral side.

Symptoms of pinch off syndrome are seen on average at 5 days with continuous infusions and 120 days with intermittent infusions (Macklin & Chernecky 2004).

Pinch off can be diagnosed using the following methods:

- Radiographic findings confirm pinch off using fluoroscopy or intravenous contrast.
- Patient should be X-rayed with their arms straight by their sides and upright, not the standard shoulder raised and rolled forward position.
- Must ascertain that PWO is not due to other cause, e.g. fibrin sheath, tip against vein wall, clot/precipitate.

The length of time from when a catheter is placed until it may fracture and embolise is variable, and the catheter fracture may be related to the degree of compression or frequency of catheter use, or both. The severity of the pinch off is assigned a grade ranging from 0 (no distortion) to 3 (catheter fracture or transaction). Catheters with grade 2 or 3 pinch off should be removed (McPhee 1999).

Signs and symptoms of catheter fracture

The following are clinical symptoms consistent with catheter fracture:

- infraclavicular pain and/or swelling, with flushing or infusion;
- palpitations;
- chest pain.
- shortness of breath
- cough

There may also be inadequate catheter length discovered after the catheter has been removed (Macklin & Chernecky 2004). Patients with catheters which are partially or completely transected will report infraclavicular pain or swelling, or both, due to infiltration or extravasation. When the catheter tip embolises patients may be asymptomatic: fewer than a third of patients have had associated symptoms.

Prevention of catheter fracture

- Adhere to the manufacturers specification for safe pressure with the device.
- Use clamps on clamping sleeves.
- Avoid using scissors or sharp objects around the catheter.
- Use short small-bore needles if accessing an injection port.
- Check patency using 10 ml or larger syringes.
- Avoid using smaller syringes wherever possible.
- Administer medication without force.
- Monitor catheters for pinholes, cuts, leaks or tears.
- Check dressing for moisture or leaking at the insertion site, during infusion and/or injection.
- Educate the patient for the signs and symptoms to look out for, and when to report.

Management

Immediate management would be to clamp the catheter and assess the degree of damage. Damaged catheters must be repaired or removed as any opening in the catheter can act as a potential entry for bacteria or air (Perdue 2001). In the case of a catheter fracture, removal of the catheter and retrieval of the fragment can be successfully carried out in interventional radiology. In the case of a PICC fracture, in order to retrieve the fragment it may be necessary to perform a venous cutdown. If the fragment has migrated then percutenous removal or a thoracotomy may be necessary (Ingle 1995).

INFECTION

Infection is one of the greatest complications associated with a central venous catheter. Bloodstream infection is the eighth leading cause of death in the USA (Hadaway 2003). The catheter provides the ideal opportunity for micro-organisms to either track along the outside of the catheter, or be administered, via the hub, internally into the central venous system. Infections can occur at the insertion site or systemically. Signs of infection at the insertion site include erythema, oedema, tracking along the length of the catheter, tenderness at the site, exudate, such as pus or an offensive smell. Septicaemia is a systemic infection which is usually characterised by pyrexia, flushing, sweating and rigors, particularly when the catheter is flushed.

Incidence

Bacteria colonising the surface of a catheter are released into the bloodstream causing bacteraemia, accounting for 6% of hospital-acquired infections and affecting 3 in every 1000 adult patients. In the critically ill this increases to 10 per 1000, and in haematology patients 6 per 1000. Intravenous devices account for at least 38% of these infections and bloodstream infections are associated with a fatality rate of at least 20%, increasing to 35% in the critically ill (Wilson 2001; CDC 2002).

Causative organisms

There are many organisms implicated in catheter related infections (see Table 8.1). The most common causative organism is *Staphylococcus*. It is a gram-positive bacteria, which is commensal flora on some parts of the body and commonly found on the skin. Some are pathogens and others have potential for

Table 8.1 Organisms implicated in catheter related infections.

Coagulase negative staphylococci	37%
Methicillin resistant *Staph. aureus*	17%
Methicillin sensitive *Staph. aureus*	14.1%
Enterococcus	6.9%
Candida	4%
Enterobacter	2.7%
Klebsiella	2.3%
E. coli	1.9%
Pseudomonas aeruginosa	1.3%
Others	12.8%

(Adapted from Kiernan 2003)

pathogenicity in the compromised host. The most common type implicated in intravenous infection is *Staphylococcus epidermidis*, a common skin commensal (Wilson 2001). It is of low virulence, but has the same attributes and ability to adhere to foreign bodies as more pathogenic *Staphylococcus*, making it difficult to treat an infected device. Other abilities that make it a significant pathogen include:

- Phagocytic and toxic shock inducing toxins.
- The production of enzyme coagulase fibrinogen into fibrin, forming a protective barrier around the invading bacteria, preventing penetration by the body's natural defences and a systemic form of treatment (Kiernan 2003).

Infection can be categorised into early (within 2–3 weeks after insertion) and delayed (more than 2–3 weeks after insertion) (Ray 1999). Early infections usually occur due to bacterial contamination during the initial insertion, are most commonly caused by skin flora, and are likely to be attributable to inadequate skin preparation or cleaning before insertion. Local infections can present as a cellulitis, adjacent to the exit site or over the port, and patients may remain afebrile throughout the course of their therapy. Delayed infections are often due to poor wound care, migration of micro-organisms along the catheter tract or seeding from a secondary source. The list of micro-organisms causing delayed infections is long and includes gram negative, positive and fungal organisms.

Sources of micro-organisms

- *Skin flora of patients or hospital staff*: resistant skin flora varies in the number of species, depending on local conditions, such as lipid production, temperature, moisture, pH and the number of hair follicles. Normal colonisation of skin at the antecubital fossa, where skin is dry and cool is approximately 10 colony forming units (cfu) per site, compared with 1000–10 000 colony forming units per site on the thorax or the neck, where lipid content and temperature are higher. These rates are altered by hospitalisation and antibiotic administration, and normal skin flora may be replaced by resistant organisms within a week (Ryder 2001). Organisms originating from the skin are predominately involved in catheter related bloodstream infections in non-tunnelled catheters and those which are in situ for short periods of time, such as less than eight days.
- *Micro-organisms which gain access to the catheter via hubs, internal lumen of catheter or external surface of catheter*: Organisms colonising the hub or port septum are predominately involved in catheter related bloodstream infections in long-term tunnelled catheters or implanted ports, and devices which are usually in situ for longer periods of time, such as more than eight days (Ryder 2001) (see Table 8.2).
- *Haematogenous seeding from a more distant source.*
- *Contaminated infusion fluids (rare).*
- *Micro-organisms which can be impacted onto the catheter distal tip at the time of insertion.* It is now suggested that bacteria are well established on surfaces of catheters which have been in situ for only one day, and that organisms from the skin can be impacted onto inserting equipment and the distal tip of the catheter as they pass through the skin during insertion (see Fig. 8.2).

Diagnosis

Many central venous catheter infections are undiagnosed, or only become recognised when septicaemia has ensued (see Table 8.3).

Table 8.2 Criteria for choosing a catheter in relation to infection risk.

- Type of vessel: venous/arterial
- Lifespan (less than 30 days, long term)
- Site of insertion (subclavian, femoral, internal jugular veins)
- Pathway from skin to vessel (tunnelled or non-tunnelled)
- Length (long, short)
- Individual characteristics (number of lumens, cuffed, impregnated)

(Reproduced with permission from Parker, L. (2002) Management of intravascular devices to prevent infection. *British Journal of Nursing*, **11**(4) 240.

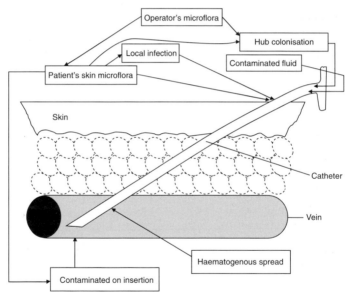

Fig. 8.2 Cross-section of the skin and underlying tissue at site of catherisation showing sources of infection in central venous access devices.

Methods for diagnosis include the following (Elliott 1998; Wilson 2001):

(1) Semi-quantitative assay, where the distal tip of the removed catheter is rolled back and forth over an agar plate. This only

Table 8.3 Criteria used for diagnosis of catheter related infection.

Local infection at skin insertion site
- erythema
- oedema
- exudate (particularly purulent)
- pain

Systemic infection/septicaemia
- low grade pyrexia
- no other obvious focus of infection
- infection unresponsive to broad spectrum antibiotics (particularly against gram negative aerobic bacillus)
- positive distal catheter tip cultures (internal and external surfaces)
- positive blood cultures taken from central venous access device and separate venepuncture, with more micro-organisms in the CVAD cultures

(Reproduced from Elliott, T. et al. (1998) Prevention of central venous catheter related infection. *Journal of Hospital Infection*, **40**, 193. With permission of Elsevier.)

samples the external surfaces and has low positive predicted value.

(2) Flushing of internal lumen of removed catheter with broth, followed by sonication (internal lumen).

(3) When catheter in situ: an intraluminal brush samples the catheter's internal surface.

(4) Acridine orange staining of blood obtained from the catheter.

(5) Blood from cultures is obtained from the catheter and separate venepuncture. This is the most widely accepted method of diagnosis.

Prevention

There are a number of recommendations related to prevention of infection, e.g. Centre for Disease Control (CDC 2002); Department of Health EPIC guidelines (DoH 2001; Pellowe et al. 2004); National Institute for Clinical Excellence (NICE 2003) and Royal College of Nursing (RCN 2003). Whilst all these guidelines and standards are developed by a multidisciplinary group of healthcare professionals, are evidence based, provide recommendations for best practice and cover a wide range of topics, there is still little known about what practitioners actually do in clinical practice. Rickard et al. (2004) found that there was inconsistent adherence to the guidelines used and there was variation in the infection control approach to CVC care. Table 8.4 illustrates that even within the guidelines there are discrepancies amongst the recommendations. Table 8.5 details interventions useful in preventing infections.

Right type of catheter material

Silicone is more likely to become contaminated with *Staphylococcus aureus*. Polyurethane coated with hydromers results in an ultra-smooth surface, which is less likely to be colonised and has led to the development of polymers containing or coated with antimicrobials. Raad et al. (1997) showed that minocycline and rifampin significantly reduced the risk of catheter related colonisation and bloodstream infections. Raad et al. (1998) repeated this finding in a second study and found the drugs inhibited ultrastructural colonisation of indwelling catheters and maintained effective activity for at least two weeks. Maki et al. (1997) found that catheters impregnated with chlorhexidine and silver sulphadiazine were well tolerated, reduced the incidence of catheter related infections and extended the time non-cuffed central venous catheters could safely be left in situ, as well as showing cost savings. Logghe et al. (1997) used the same type of catheter as Maki, but did not find an overall reduction in risk of bloodstream infections in haematology patients.

Safest insertion site

It has been shown that the femoral vein is associated with the highest rate of infections and the subclavian vein the lowest (Pellowe et al. 2004). However, using the peripheral route for central venous access, e.g. PICC, has a lower rate than the chest. (Elliott 1998; DoH 2001; Wilson 2001; CDC 2002).

Correct antiseptic agents to prepare site

As the skin is the major source of micro-organisms which contaminate the catheter the use of correct antiseptic is vital. The main types are 2% chlorhexidine, 10% povidone iodine and 70%

Table 8.4 Recommendations of all main organisations.

Recommendations	DoH 2001 (EPIC)	CDC 2002	NICE 2003	RCN 2003	Pellowe et al. 2004 (EPIC)
Catheter lumen: use single unless multiple are essential, especially for TPN.	✓	✓	✓	✓	
Consider the use of an antimicrobial impregnated catheter for adults who require short-term catheterisation and are at high risk of infection.	✓	✓		✓	✓
Unless medically contra-indicated, use subclavian site in preference to jugular/femoral site for non-tunnelled catheter, and consider use of PICC instead of subclavian or jugular.	✓	✓			✓
Use optimum aseptic technique during catheter placement, i.e. sterile gown, sterile gloves and large sterile drapes.	✓	✓	✓	✓	✓
Prepare insertion site using alcoholic chlorhexidine gluconate and allow it to dry.	✓	✓		✓	✓
Do not routinely apply antimicrobial ointment.	✓	✓			
Disinfect external surfaces of catheter hub and connection ports with chlorhexidine, unless contra-indicated.	✓	✓	✓	✓	✓

Continued

Table 8.4 *Continued.*

Recommendations	DoH 2001 (EPIC)	CDC 2002	NICE 2003	RCN 2003	Pellowe et al. 2004 (EPIC)
Use semi-permeable transparent dressing and replace every seven days or when it becomes damp, soiled or loosened.	✓	✓	✓	✓	
Use sterile gauze if patient is sweating profusely, or the site is bleeding or oozing, and change daily or replace when it becomes damp, soiled or loosened.	✓		✓	✓	
Routinely flush open-ended catheters with anticoagulant to prevent catheter thrombus (unless advised otherwise).	✓	✓	✓	✓	✓
Do not routinely replace non-tunnelled CVC. Use guidewire exchange to replace malfunctioning catheter if there is no evidence of infection.	✓	✓			
Replace intravenous administration set when device replaced, no more frequently than 72 hours, unless clinically indicated or if TPN infused.	✓	✓	✓	✓	
Antibiotic prophylaxis unnecessary.	✓	✓	✓		
In-line filters should not be routinely used.		✓	✓		
Promote use of needleless systems whenever possible.		✓	✓	✓	

Table 8.5 Interventions to reduce the risk of infection.

- right type of catheter material
- safest insertion site
- optimum aseptic technique on insertion
- right antiseptic agents to prepare site
- correct technique and antiseptic to care for catheter and site
- correct catheter replacement strategy
- antibiotic policy only when indicated

alcohol. Maki et al. (1991) found chlorhexidine to be the best cleaning solution and this is supported by Pellowe et al. (2004).

Correct technique and antiseptic to care for catheter and site

The site should be monitored at least daily for the presence of signs and symptoms of complications. The dressing should be changed regularly and the correct dressing used, usually a transparent dressing or gauze. Antibiotic ointments have been used successfully, but do increase the risk of acquiring a catheter related infection caused by candida. Mupirocin resistance has also been reported so use is limited (CDC 2002). It is also important to keep access points and catheter lumens to a minimum and these should be cleaned properly.

Colonisation of connectors and hubs are an important source of micro-organisms in the development of sepsis. If a strict aseptic technique is not adhered to during manipulations, sites could become contaminated and act as a potential source for systemic contamination. In one study in an ITU setting, 22% of stopcocks were shown to be contaminated with micro-organisms within 72 hours (Tebbs et al. 1995). Use of needleless connectors acts as a barrier to micro-organisms, as well as reducing the likelihood of needlestick injury, but still need to be cleaned. It is now recommended that administration sets are changed every 72 hours when used for continuous infusions of solutions, but may need changing more frequently if used for intermittent infusions, blood or lipids (NICE 2003; RCN 2003). In-line filters have been used to prevent infections developing due to contaminated infusion fluids and to inhibit debris entering the catheter, which encourages thrombus formation and infection. If used, they need to be changed frequently and this may increase the number of manipulations and cost, but they are not recommended for routine use.

Flushing and maintaining patency is vital to reduce the development of thrombus and possible colonisation. Daily flushing with heparin and vancomycin has been shown to significantly reduce catheter related sepsis compared to heparin alone, but widespread use of antibiotics may encourage vancomycin resistant gram negative cocci (CDC 2002).

Correct catheter replacement strategy

The risk of catheter related infections increases with the duration of the catheter. There are no universally accepted standard guidelines for optimum changing time for CVCs. Practices range from 3–4 days, to only when sepsis becomes evident. It is also common to leave the catheter for as long as possible, but monitor the patient closely. If a catheter related infection develops, the catheter should be removed and replaced at a different site. If removal is as a result of malfunction then the catheter may be exchanged over a guidewire, although this can increase the risk of infection and should not be performed if the patient has any signs or symptoms of infection (RCN 2003).

Antibiotic policy only when indicated

Prophylactic antibiotics given just before insertion appear to be of no benefit in preventing catheter infections (CDC 2002).

Management

Course of action depends on (Ray 1999):

(1) patient factors;
(2) type of organism involved;
(3) need for CVAD;
(4) type of infection.

The immune status should be assessed, as it will determine the aggressiveness of treatment. In patients with a normal immune status catheter salvage should be considered as the main aim of therapy. In patients with severe compromised immune status, protecting the patients from a progressive infection must be the primary goal. Other factors include virulence of micro-organisms, determined not just by culture of the site or lumen but by clinical advancement of the infectious process. If infection progresses very rapidly clinically then more aggressive therapy needs to be initiated. The type of infection, e.g. local or systemic also determines the type of therapy.

Local infection is usually treated with antibiotics given orally or intravenously and sometimes topically. Tunnel or port infections are treated in the same way unless there is an abscess in the pocket, which may necessitate the removal of the device and drainage of the area. Systemic infection is often treated with intravenous antibiotics or oral and intravenous antibiotics. If there is evidence of a fibrin sheath then concomitant urokinase administration and antibiotics therapy may prove more effective. Thrombolytic agents break down fibrin and exposes the micro-organisms to the antibiotics administered via the lumen. In the case of septic thrombo-phlebitis the treatment is removal of the catheter and administration of intravenous antibiotics.

THROMBOSIS
A thrombosis is a clot of blood that can be present at the tip of a catheter or can surround the catheter, for example a thrombosis in the upper arm caused by the presence of a PICC. The cause is usually multi-factorial (Wickham et al. 1992; Mayo 2000). Venous thrombi consist mainly of fibrin and tightly bound red blood cells. They are large, with tapering tails that extend into larger veins, and are attached to the venous intima, usually at a valve or bifurcation.

An SVC thrombus is when a catheter chronically rubs against the wall of the SVC. It provokes thrombosis at the site and is often associated with a fibrin sheath. If the thrombus becomes large enough to obstruct blood flow, symptoms may develop including suffusion, fullness in head and neck, blurred vision and vertigo (Perdue 2001).

Incidence
The literature varies as to the exact incidence of catheter related thrombosis, covering ranges from 3–79% (Moureau et al. 1999),

with ultrasound studies showing an incidence of 33–67% after more than one week (and about 40% at autopsy; Galloway & Bodenham 2004). However, clinical rates are low, particularly in long-term access, and asymptomatic subclavian vein thrombosis is more common, with only 1–5% demonstrating symptoms (Moureau et al. 1999).

Causes/predisposing factors
In order for a thrombosis to develop it requires three factors (Mayo 2001; Perdue 2001), and is known as Vichow's triad:

(1) stasis;
(2) endothelial damage;
(3) hypercoagable state (caused by the following conditions: diabetes, malnutrition, dehydration, pregnancy, osteomyelitis, smoking, chronic renal failure, cirrhosis, cancer, obesity, sickle cell, surgery, congestive heart failure, oestrogen therapies).

There are certain groups of patients who are at a greater risk of developing a thrombosis (Perdue 2001):

- patients with malignancy, especially lung cancer and lymphoma;
- venous compression by tumour metastases;
- inflammatory bowel syndrome;
- hyper-coaguability;
- infusion of sclerosing agents;
- improper maintenance;
- sepsis.

Signs and symptoms
Symptoms can be very acute or vague. The patient will usually complain of pain in the area, such as the arm or the neck, and oedema of the neck, chest and upper extremity. There may also be periorbital oedema, facial tenderness, tachycardia, shortness of breath and sometimes a cough, signs of a collateral circulation over the chest area, jugular venous distension and discolouration of the limb (Perdue 2001).

Prevention

Mayo (2000) outlines the main preventative measures:

- Correct placement of tip in the SVC.
- Constant assessment of function while the catheter is in situ.
- Early intervention with a thrombolytic agent.
- Meticulous flushing with pulsatile positive pressure flush.

Tip placement is associated with the incidence of thrombosis. It has been found that catheters whose tips lie in the axillary, subclavian or brachiocephalic veins have a greater incidence of thrombosis (Moureau et al. 1999; Vesely 2003). This is reduced by placing the tip into the lower third of the SVC or into the right atrium. The reason for this is that the blood flow is greater and the vessel larger; therefore there is less trauma and rubbing of the catheter against the vein wall. Left-sided placement, particularly of PICCs, has also been associated with greater risk. This could be related to the tip position when placed in the left side (Moureau et al. 1999; Perdue 2001). The skill of the practitioners may also have an impact, as it has been noted that when first learning to insert PICCs, the rate of thrombosis is higher and this could be related to the amount of time taken to insert and trauma caused on insertion (Perdue 2001).

It is still unclear whether the addition of an anticoagulant whilst the catheter is in situ makes any difference to the incidence of thrombosis in all patients. Lokich & Becker (1983) found that the administration of 1 mg warfarin daily during the period a long-term access device, such as a tunnelled catheter, was in situ appeared to reduce the risk. Bern et al. (1990) showed that in patients with long-term CVCs who were randomised into requiring 1 mg of warfarin or not, given 3 days prior to insertion and continuing for 90 days, it can protect against thrombosis without inducing a haemorrhagic state. Patients who are at a greater risk of thrombosis may need to be fully anticoagulated and have regular blood checks performed to check their clotting screen. However, there are those who feel that warfarin is unnecessary. In a study of 1589 patients, comparing those taking warfarin with a control group, and those taking dose-adjusted warfarin (DAW) with warfarin 1 mg, Young et al. (2005) concluded that there is no apparent benefit in using low-dose warfarin for prophylaxis of symptomatic CVC-related thrombosis in patients with cancer. They also concluded that if clinicians chose to offer prophylaxis, DAW would be superior but at the cost of increased risk of bleeding. Couban et al. (2005) also found that warfarin had no effect on CVC lifespan or on the number of premature CVC removals or frequency of major bleeding episodes in patients with cancer.

Management
The patient should have a venogram and ultrasound to diagnose the thrombosis (Perdue 2001). Treatment can be either catheter removal or anticoagulation, as thrombolytic therapy has proved successful in extreme cases and is often dependent on the size of the clot and area of impaired circulation (Perdue 2001). Pharmacological management of thrombosis includes:

(1) Anticoagulants: intravenous heparin acts to impair blood coagulation by neutralising several clotting factors. It does not assist in lysis of formed clots but reduces the occurrence. The main side effect is haemorrhage.
(2) Thrombolytics contain enzymes, which convert plasminogen into plasmin and result in lysis of the clot. Urokinase serum has a half-life of approximately 20 minutes (Moureau et al. 1999; Perdue 2001).

If the catheter is to be removed, patients will be prescribed heparin, and this may continue for a number of days before they are switched onto an oral anticoagulant, such as warfarin. This may then need to continue for up to three months following removal.

CATHETER OCCLUSION
Before effective interventions 25% of all catheters placed were removed due to catheter related occlusions. Of these, 58% were thrombotic and 42% non-thrombotic/mechanical (Andris & Krzywda 1997b). Catheters may become occluded for a number of reasons:

(1) blood clot within the lumen;
(2) fibrin sheath/tail;
(3) precipitation of drugs.

There are two main types of occlusion: persistent withdrawal occlusion and total occlusion. Persistent withdrawal occlusion (PWO) is when the catheter will flush, but will not enable the practitioner to withdraw blood, which may affect the ability to gain a sample and, more importantly, may prevent the practitioner from checking patency of the device (Mayo 2001). Total occlusion is when there is an inability to withdraw blood and infuse or inject into the catheter (Mayo 2001).

Thrombotic occlusions

Types
There are many types of thrombotic occlusions:

(1) Intraluminal thrombus (see Fig. 8.3a)
    These occur as partial occlusions and account for 5–25% of all catheter occlusion (Krzydwa 1999). They usually result from:
    (a) insufficient or poor technique when flushing (i.e. not using positive pressure);
    (b) inadequate flow through lumens of the catheter; allowing an infusion to run dry, which allows blood to track back up the tubing, or switching off of an infusion without flushing;
    (c) reflux from changes in intra-thoracic pressure, coughing, congestive heart failure, heavy lifting, frequent withdrawal of blood via catheter.
    These may cause sluggish flow, apparent on flushing or infusing solutions (Haire & Herbst 2000).

(2) Fibrin tail (flap) (see Fig. 8.3b)
    This occurs when fibrin, blood cells and platelets adhere to the end of the catheter. Tails become quite long as more cells and other blood products are deposited progressively on the tail. The inability to withdraw blood is frequently caused by the tail. PWO that acts as a one-way valve allows the catheter to flush, but doesn't allow blood to be aspirated (Haire & Herbst 2000).

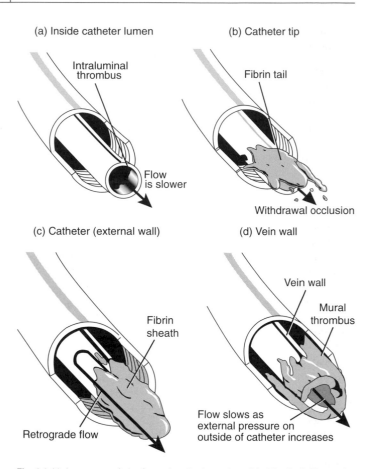

(a) Inside catheter lumen

Intraluminal thrombus

Flow is slower

(b) Catheter tip

Fibrin tail

Withdrawal occlusion

(c) Catheter (external wall)

Fibrin sheath

Retrograde flow

(d) Vein wall

Vein wall

Mural thrombus

Flow slows as external pressure on outside of catheter increases

Fig. 8.3 Various types of clot formation. Redrawn from Macklin, D. & Chernecky, C. (2004) *IV Therapy*. Saunders, St Louis. With permission of Elsevier.

(3) Fibrin sheath (sleeve) (see Fig. 8.3c)

This is extraluminal, occurring when fibrin adheres to the external surface of the catheter. A fibrin sleeve may resemble a sock and encase the whole catheter at the tip, and this may extend along the entire catheter to the point where the catheter exits onto the skin. It can develop in the majority of silicone catheters in as little as 48 hours, or up to several months after placement (Wickham et al. 1992; Mayo 2000).

The consequences of fibrin sheaths are:

(a) elimination of an important catheter function, such as blood withdrawal or drug administration;

(b) can be seeded with bacteria, and micro-organisms can then be disseminated into bloodstream when the catheter is flushed, or during checking for blood return;

(c) drug extravasation: fibrin deposits can encase the entire catheter and there is then a potential risk of fluid backtracking along the outside portion and exiting out of the venous entry site and into the chest wall (Mayo 2000).

(4) Mural thrombus (see Fig. 8.3d)

If the catheter tip causes a vessel wall injury, a mural thrombosis may form, as the fibrin from the vessel wall injury attracts to the fibrin building on the catheter surface. Whilst it is not significant in itself it can increase the potential risk of venous thrombosis from 0.7–74%.

Incidence

The incidence of thrombotic catheter dysfunction is between 3–7%. It depends on the type of illness, type of catheter and duration of catheter in situ. The risk is increased if the tip is high in the SVC and innominate vein (incidence 75%). In post-mortem 97% show fibrin sheath in place within less than a week. In oncology patients with CVADs, 62% of catheters had complications and 30% had fibrin tails (Moureau et al. 1999).

Non-thrombotic occlusion

These account for 5% of all catheter occlusions (Moureau et al. 1999). Causes can be:

• simple mechanical, external clamps;
• kinking of catheter;
• constricting sutures;
• dislodged needles;
• pinch off syndrome (which causes it in 1.1% of patients);
• precipitation.

Intraluminal precipitates

Mixing of incompatible medications within the catheter lumen can often lead to precipitation and occlusion. This may occur when drugs are not flushed adequately. Solubility is highly dependent on drug concentration and pH. Intravenous lipid, calcium salts and phosphate complexes, as well as antibiotics, can all result in precipitate formation. Lipid occlusion may slowly accumulate within the catheter lumen, presenting as resistance to flushing over several days before complete occlusion.

Diagnosis

Steps in catheter occlusion assessment include:

- Catheter function, infusion/blood aspiration.
- External occlusion, kinking/clamps, etc.
- Postural changes: if relieved when position changed.
- Relevant catheter use: history of what was infused, blood products, aspiration.
- Physical assessment: assess patients for signs of oedema, redness, pain or dilated vessels.

Pinch off syndrome can be diagnosed with a chest X-ray, and fibrin sleeves by injection of contrast. A Doppler ultrasound can diagnose a thrombosis, and a venogram is usually used for diagnosing an SVC thrombosis (Krzywda 1999; Simcock 2001).

Prevention

Effective flushing is the key to prevention: flushing between drugs, flushing using the correct solution, in the correct volume and at the correct frequency, using the correct technique, will reduce the risk of occlusion. Ensuring that infusions which are infused via a volumetric pump have a KVO (keep vein open) facility to prevent backflow, and that infusion bags are changed as soon as necessary, all help to reduce the risk. Injection caps which enable positive displacement may also be of benefit, as well as using valved catheters.

Management

The first step to management is to ascertain the cause of the occlusion. Once the practitioner has ascertained the cause they can then follow the algorithm (see Fig. 8.4) where appropriate.

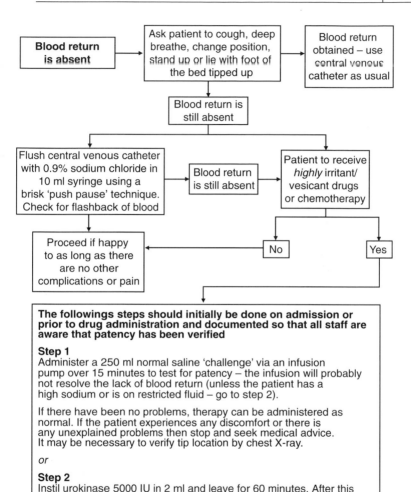

The followings steps should initially be done on admission or prior to drug administration and documented so that all staff are aware that patency has been verified

Step 1

Administer a 250 ml normal saline 'challenge' via an infusion pump over 15 minutes to test for patency – the infusion will probably not resolve the lack of blood return (unless the patient has a high sodium or is on restricted fluid – go to step 2).

If there have been no problems, therapy can be administered as normal. If the patient experiences any discomfort or there is any unexplained problems then stop and seek medical advice. It may be necessary to verify tip location by chest X-ray.

or

Step 2

Instil urokinase 5000 IU in 2 ml and leave for 60 minutes. After this time withdraw the urokinase and assess the catheter again. Repeat as necessary. If blood return is still absent, it may be necessary to verify tip location by chest X-ray.

Fig. 8.4 Algorithm for persistent withdrawal occlusion. (Adapted from UCL Hospital Central Venous Catheter Policy.)

Drug precipitation

There are a number of agents that can be used to help dissolve drug or lipid precipitation. Choice of a pharmacological agent is based on suspected history of occlusion (Reed & Philips 1996). Examples include: 3 ml of 7% alcohol for unblocking occusions caused by lipids and 0.1 N hydrochloric acid for antibiotics.

Thrombotic occlusions

In the case of a blood clot or fibrin causing the occlusion, the solution of choice is a fibrinolytic agent. Urokinase works by breaking down fibrin and thereby dissolving the clot. It has been used effectively for years in the UK for both PWO and total occlusions. The usual dose is 5000 iu in 2 ml of water for injection instilled into the catheter lumen and left for 1–2 hours. Anecdotally, practitioners have found it more effective if left for longer periods of time, even over 24 hours, although the potency of the drug decreases over time. Another alternative to urokinase is alteplase. Ponec et al. (2001) found that alteplase 2 mg per 2 ml was effective at restoring flow in catheters. After two hour's treatment, function was restored to 74% of devices instilled with alteplase and only 17% with placebo. After a 1–2 hour treatment, 90% function was resolved and no serious drug related adverse events were documented, leading to the conclusion that it was safe and effective. This was also supported by work carried out by Dietcher (2002) and Timoney et al. (2002).

One of the key factors in unblocking a catheter is to use a technique which does not create extra pressure within the lumen, as this may result in damage to the catheter. Conn (1993) advocated the use of a 10 ml, or larger, syringe when flushing or unblocking a central venous catheter and this is because of the pressure created by smaller syringes. The unit of measurement used for pressure generated by a syringe is psi or pounds per square inch. A 1 ml syringe used on an occluded catheter can create up to 150 psi. It only takes 35 psi to pump up a car tyre! As a result, a technique was devised that enabled the fibrinolytic drug to be instilled without creating unnecessary pressure, called the negative pressure technique. A three-way tap is used so that a vacuum is created along one section, and then, when the tap is turned towards the solution it is 'sucked' in

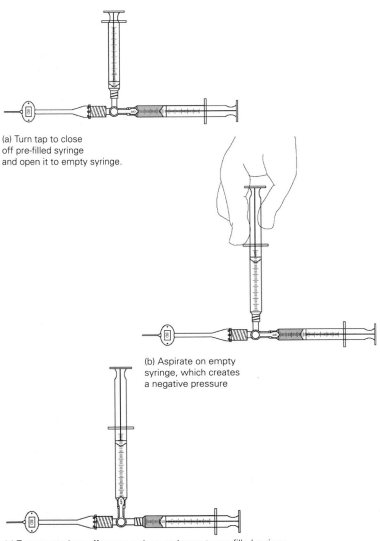

(a) Turn tap to close
off pre-filled syringe
and open it to empty syringe.

(b) Aspirate on empty
syringe, which creates
a negative pressure

(c) Turn tap to close off empty syringe and open to pre-filled syringe.
The medication will automatically be aspirated into the catheter. Repeat as necessary.

Fig. 8.5 Unblocking an occluded catheter. (Adapted from BD First PICC Clinical Education Class Manual D11952B 5/98.)

without any undue pressure (Krzywda 1999; Moureau et al. 1999; Dougherty 2004; Gabriel 2004) (see Fig. 8.5).

Fibrin sheaths may require mechanical stripping with a wire. The procedure is usually performed by an interventional radiologist, who advances a snare through the femoral vein and loops it around the catheter, pulling down on the shaft of the catheter while applying traction, thus removing the fibrin (Krzywda 1999). Complications include possible fracture of the catheter, embolism and infection, but the techniques in one study have shown that patency was restored initially in 98% of catheters and with 54% at three months (Crain et al. 1996). Endoluminal brushes (Archis et al. 2000) can be used to declot various types of CVC. In a study of dialysis catheters that were totally occluded or produced flows inadequate for dialysis, endoluminal brushing (with or without additional urokinase) resolved patency in 42% of catheters and the data suggests a role for using the brushes in early management, as no complications were shown.

EXTRAVASATION

Extravasation is the inadvertent administration of vesicant drugs into surrounding tissues, which can lead to tissue necrosis (How & Brown 1998; Weinstein 2001; RCN 2003; Dougherty 2004). A vesicant is any drug which has the potential to cause tissue damage and require some form of management (see Fig. 8.6).

Outcomes of CVAD extravasation include (Hyde 2004):

- sloughing of tissues;
- pain;
- infection;
- loss of mobility of extremity;
- amputation/major surgical procedures;
- litigation.

Incidence

CVADs are devices of choice for patients receiving infusions of cytotoxic drugs and/or vesicant medications. The actual number of CVAD extravasations is unknown, although 6% of port extravasations are due to needle dislodgement (Schulmeister & Camp Sorrell 2000; Lawson 2003; Masoorli 2003).

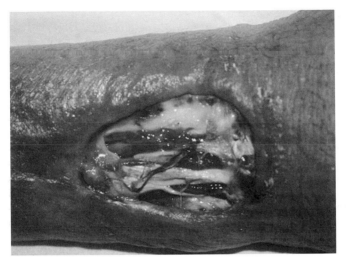

Fig. 8.6 Injury as a result of extravasation.

Causes

Causes of extravasation include (Schulmeister 1989, 1998; Mayo 1998):

- catheter tip malposition;
- catheter malfunction;
- internal catheter fracture/catheter/port separation;
- incorrect port access/needle placement;
- needle dislodgement;
- thrombus or fibrin sheath formation;
- faulty equipment;
- human error;
- system problems.

Drugs capable of causing tissue necrosis

There are a number of drugs which have the potential to cause tissue damage for a number of reasons, e.g. vesicant, pH, osmolarity. The following are some examples:

- Non-cytotoxic drugs such as:
  Calcium gluconate and chloride, phenytoin, any hypertonic solutions, e.g. sodium bicarbonate (greater than 5%) or dextrose (greater than 10%), amphotericin, aciclovir, diazepam, digoxin, ganciclovir, potassium chloride (if greater than 40 mmol/l).
- Cytotoxic drugs such as:
  Vinca alkaloids, carmustine (concentrated solution), dacarbazine (concentrated solution), doxorubicin, epirubicin, mitomycin C.

Drugs should not be reconstituted to give solutions which are higher than the manufacturer's recommended concentration, and the method of administration should be checked, e.g. infusion, injection. Drug data sheets should always be checked and the pharmacy departments should be consulted if the information is insufficient.

Signs and symptoms

Extravasation should be suspected if (Hyde 2004):

- The patient complains of burning, stinging pain or any other acute change at the catheter insertion site or anywhere along the path of the catheter, e.g. along the tunnel.
- Swelling or leakage occurs at the catheter insertion site, or if there is any swelling along the tunnel site.
- If no blood return is obtained when the plunger of the syringe is pulled back, this may indicate lack of patency and incorrect position of device. Any change in blood flow should be investigated.
- A resistance is felt on the plunger of the syringe if drugs are given by bolus.
- There is absence of free flow when administration is by infusion.

Note: One or more of the above may be present. Any extravasation from a port is problematic due to the depth of a port and slower development of demonstrable signs. Therefore, if extravasation is suspected, or once confirmed, action must be taken immediately (Weinstein 2001).

Prevention
Check tip verification by:

- Checking blood return.
- Correct needle placement in ports: ensure backplate of port is felt and there is free flowing blood return.

Management
The management of the extravasation of chemotherapeutic agents is controversial. There is little documented evidence of efficacy, especially in relation to extravasation from CVADs. Controlled clinical trials are lacking and it is often difficult to ascertain whether an extravasation has actually occurred (Weinstein 2001; Hyde 2004). The general management of extravasation involves several stages, but not all these can be related to the management of CVAD extravasation.

Stopping the injection and withdrawing (aspirating) the drug
Some authors recommend the withdrawal of as much of the drug as possible, as soon as extravasation is suspected, as this may help to reduce the size of the lesion, but it can only be performed during a bolus injection, not an infusion (Oncology Nursing Society 1999; Weinstein 2001; Hyde 2004).

Immediate removal of the device
This is usually not practical with a CVAD (except with a PICC), and may only be performed once the extravasation has been confirmed, and may require medical intervention.

Applying hot or cold packs
These packs could be applied to the area where the extravasation is suspected, but there is no evidence that they will be effective. Cold packs are used to cause vasoconstriction, which reduces the local destructive effect by reducing local uptake of the drug by the tissues, reducing local oedema and slowing metabolic rates of the cells (Hyde 2004). The time suggested for application ranges from 15 minutes 4 times a

day (Rudolph & Larson 1987) to every 20–40 minutes for 24–48 hours. Hot packs are recommended specifically for the management of non-DNA binding drugs, such as vinca alkaloids. It is used to increase blood supply and increase dispersion and absorption of the neutralising agent (Hyde 2004). The increase in blood supply may also help promote healing (Weinstein 2001). It is recommended that the pack be applied for 15–20 minutes, four times a day for 24–48 hours. However, this may be difficult for nurses and/or patients to comply with, depending on where the CVAD is located.

Use of antidotes

There are a number of antidotes available, but again there is a lack of scientific evidence to demonstrate their value. There appear to be two main types: one is used to dilute the drug, e.g. hyaluronidase, and the other to neutralise the drugs and reduce inflammation, e.g. steroids (Stanley 2002; Hyde 2004). Hyaluronidase is an enzyme which destroys tissue cement, aiding in reducing or preventing tissue damage by allowing rapid diffusion of the extravasated fluid and promoting drug absorption. The usual dose is 1500 iu. The evidence regarding the use of steroids is that it is of no benefit at all. DMSO (a topical solution) has been shown to be effective in reducing damage following anthracycline extravasations (How & Brown 1998).

Surgery

In the case of CVAD extravasation, a referral to a plastic surgeon is crucial to limit the degree of damage. It may be necessary to remove the tissue containing the drug, thereby removing the damaging effects, which can continue whilst the drug remains in situ. Requirement for surgery is usually based upon the size and location of the extravasation as well as the type of drug that has extravasated (Heckler 1989). The use of saline flushing conducted within the first 24 hours has been suggested as a less traumatic and cheaper procedure than surgery (Gault 1993). The saline flush-out technique involves four small stab incisions, which facilitates cleansing of any drug from the subcutaneous tissues and is advocated for use with DNA binding vesicants such as doxorubicin (How & Brown 1998).

The use of extravasation kits has been recommended (Hyde 2004). Kits should be assembled according to the particular needs of individual institutions. They should be kept in all areas where vesicant drugs are administered, so that staff have immediate access to equipment (Hyde 2004). The kit should be simple, to avoid confusion, but comprehensive enough to meet all reasonable needs (Stanley 2002). Instructions should be clear and easy to follow and the use of a flow chart enables staff to follow the management process.

Documentation

Any extravasation must be reported and fully documented as it is an accident and the patient will require follow-up care. Information may also be used for statistical purposes, e.g. collation and analysis using the green card scheme developed by St Chads Hospital, Birmingham. Finally, it may be required in case of litigation (Stanley 2002).

Patient information

Patients must understand the possibility of an extravasation occurring and the importance of reporting early signs and symptoms. This is important, as patients may be receiving their therapy at home and not be immediately accessible to staff. Patients should always be informed when an extravasation has occurred and be given an explanation of what has happened and what management has been carried out (McCaffrey Boyle & Engelking 1995; Hyde 2004). An information sheet should be given to patients, with instructions of what symptoms to look out for and when to contact the hospital during the follow-up period (Hyde 2004).

Legal issues

Extravasation associated with the use of CVADs often results in litigation due to the injuries caused, which can be clinically, cosmetically and psychologically damaging to the patient. Patients may hold the view that the injury was caused by the nurse's negligence, so informing the patient of the possible consequences of administration of vesicant agents is important (Dougherty 2003; Lawson 2003; Masoorli 2003).

Scenario

Sam King, aged 53, attends her local chemotherapy clinic for an infusion of pamidronate every three weeks. She has had a port in situ for over a year and never had any problems, but at her last three visits, the infusion only ran when she moved her arm out to the side. Now, she needs to start a new vesicant chemotherapy and the nurse cannot obtain any blood from the port.

What could the cause of these symptoms be and what course of action should be taken by the nurse?

These are classic symptoms of pinch off syndrome. The nurse should inform the doctor, who will probably order a X-ray and/or a cathetergram. It may be that a pinched off section can be seen on the X-ray, but this alone will not indicate if the catheter is damaged. If there is damage then when dye is injected through the catheter it will be seen leaking from the area of damage. The device will then need to be removed to prevent a catheter embolism occurring.

CONCLUSION

If the correct care and management is followed then most of the complications described in this chapter will not occur. Poor care results in the patient having a poor or non-functioning device and may even necessitate removal of the device. This results in the patient having to undergo a further invasive procedure that should be prevented at all costs.

REFERENCES

Andris, D.A. & Krzywda, E.A. (1997a) Catheter pinch off syndrome: recognition and management. *Journal of Intravenous Nursing*, **20** (5), 233–237.

Andris, D.A. & Krzywda, E.A. (1997b) Central venous access: clinical practice issues. *Nursing Clinics in North America*, **32**, 717–740.

Archis, C.A., Black, J. & Brown, M.A. (2000) Does an endoluminal catheter brush improve flows or unblock haemodialysis catheters? *Nephrology*, **5**, 55–58.

Bern, M.M., Lokich, J.J., Wallah, S.E., Bothe, A., Benotti, P.N., Arkin, C.F., Greco, F.A., Huberman, M. & Moore, C. (1990) Very low doses of warfarin can prevent thrombosis in central venous catheters: a randomised prospective trial. *Annals of Internal Medicine*, **112** (6), 423–428.

Center for Disease Control (2002) Guidelines for the prevention of intravascular catheter related infections. *Morbidity and Mortality Weekly Report*, **51** (RR10), 1–26.

Conn, C. (1993) The importance of syringe size when using an implanted vascular access device. *Journal of Vascular Access Networks*, **3** (1), 11–18.

Couban, S., Goodyear, M., Burnell, M., Dean, S., Wasi, P., Barnes, D., MacLeod, D., Burton, E., Andreou, P. & Anderson, D.R. (2005) Randomised placebo-controlled study of low-dose warfarin for the prevention of CVC-associated thrombosis in patients with cancer. *Journal of Clinical Oncology*, **23** (18), 4063–4069.

Crain, M.R., Mewissen, M.W. & Ostrowski, G.J. (1996) Fibrin sleeve stripping for salvage of failing haemodialysis: technique and initial results. *Radiology*, **198**, 41–44.

Department of Health (2001) Guidelines for preventing infections associated with the insertion and maintenance of central venous catheters. *Journal of Hospital Infection*, **47** (supplement), S47–S67.

Dietcher, S.R., Fesen, M.R., Kiproff, P.M., Hill, P.A., Li, X., McCluskey, E.R. & Samba, C.P. (2002) Safety and efficacy of alteplase for restoring function in occluded central venous catheters: results of the cardiovascular thrombolytic to open occluded lines trial. *Journal of Clinical Oncology*, **20** (1), 317–324.

Dougherty, L. (2003) The expert witness working within the legal system of the UK. *Journal of Vascular Access Devices*, **8** (2), 29–37.

Dougherty, L. (2004) Vascular access devices. In: Dougherty, L. & Lister, S. (eds) *Manual of Clinical Nursing Procedures*, 6th edn. Blackwell Science, Oxford.

Drewett, S. (2000) Complications of central venous catheters: nursing care. *British Journal of Nursing*, **9** (8), 466–478.

Elliott, T.S.J. (1993) Line associated bacteraemias. *Public Health Laboratories Service Communicable Disease Report*, **3** (7), R91–R96.

Elliott, T.S.J. et al. (1998) Prevention of central venous catheter related infection. *Journal of Hospital Infection*, **40**, 193–201.

Gabriel, J. (2004) Long-term central venous access. In: Dougherty, L. & Lamb, J. (eds) *Intravenous Therapy in Nursing Practice*. Churchill Livingstone, Edinburgh.

Galloway, S. & Bodenham, A. (2004) Long-term central venous access. *British Journal of Anaesthesia*, **92**, 722–734.

Gault, D.T. (1993) Extravasation injuries. *British Journal of Plastic Surgery*, **46** (2), 91–96.

Hadaway, L.C. (2003) Skin flora and infection. *Journal of Intravenous Nursing*, **26** (1), 44–48.

Haire, D.W. & Herbst, S.F. (2000) Use of alteplase. *Journal of Vascular Access Devices*, **5** (2), 28–36.

Heckler, F.R. (1989) Current thoughts on extravasation injuries. *Clinical Plastic Surgery*, **16** (3), 557–563.

How, C. & Brown, J. (1998) Extravasation of cytotoxic chemotherapy. *European Journal of Oncology Nursing*, **2** (1), 51–58.

Hyde, L. (2004) Drug administration: cytotoxic drugs. In: Dougherty, L. & Lister, S. (eds) *The Royal Marsden Hospital Manual of Clinical Nursing Procedures*, 6th edn, pp. 228–256. Blackwell Publishing, Oxford.

Ingle, R.J. (1995) Rare complications of vascular access devices. *Seminars in Oncology Nursing*, **11** (3), 184–193.

Kaufman, J.A. (2001) The interventional radiologist's role in providing and maintaining long-term central venous catheters. *Journal of Intravenous Nursing*, **24** (35), S23–S27.

Kiernan, M. (2003) Reducing the risks of device-related infection caused by staphylococci. *Professional Nurse*, **18** (8), 441–444.

Krzywda, E.D. (1999) Predisposing factors, prevention and management of central venous catheter occlusions. *Journal of Intravenous Nursing*, **22** (supplement), S11–S17.

Lawson, T. (2003) A legal perspective on CVC-related extravasation. *Journal of Vascular Access Devices*, (Spring), 25–27.

Logghe, C., Van Ossel, Ch., D'Hoore, W., Ezzedine, H., Wauters, G. & Haxhe, J.J. (1997) Evaluation of chlorhexidine and silversulfadiazine impregnated central venous catheters for the prevention of bloodstream infection in leukaemic patients: a randomised controlled trial. *Journal of Hospital Infection*, (37), 145–156.

Lokich, J.J. & Becker, B. (1983) Subclavian vein thrombosis in patients treated with infusion therapy for advanced malignancy. *Cancer*, **52**, 1586–1589.

McCaffrey Boyle, D. & Engelking, C. (1995) Vesicant extravasation: myths and realities. *Oncology Nursing Forum*, **22** (1), 57–65.

McGee, D.C. & Gould, M.K. (2003) Preventing complications of central venous catheterisation. *Medical Journals*, **348** (12), 1123–1133.

Macklin, D. & Chernecky, C. (2004) *Real World Nursing Survival Guide: IV Therapy*. Saunders, St. Louis.

Maki, D.G. & Ringer, M. (1987) Evaluation of dressing regimes for prevention of infection with peripheral intravenous catheters. *Journal of American Medical Association*, **258** (17), 2396–2403.

Maki, D.G., Ringer, M. & Alvarado, C.J. (1991) Prospective randomised trial of povidone-iodine alcohol and chlorhexidine for prevention of infection associated with central venous and arterial catheters. *The Lancet*, **338**, 339–343.

Maki, D.G., Stolz, S.M., Wheeler, S. & Mermel, L.A. (1997) Prevention of central venous catheter-related bloodstream infection by use of an antiseptic impregnated catheter. *Annals of Internal Medicine*, **127** (4), 257–266.

Masoorli, S. (2003) Extravasation injuries associated with the use of central vascular access devices. *Journal of Vascular Access Devices*, (Spring), 21–23.

Mayo, D.J. (1995) Chemotherapy extravasation: a consequence of fibrin sheath formation around venous access devices. *Oncology Nursing Forum*, **22** (4), 675–680.

Mayo, D.J. (1998) Fibrin sheath formation and chemotherapy extravasation: a case report. *Supportive Care in Cancer*, **6**, 51–56.

Mayo, D.J. (2000) Catheter-related thrombosis. *Journal of Vascular Access Devices*, **5** (2), 10–20.

Mayo, D.J. (2001) Catheter related thrombosis. *Journal of Intravenous Nursing*, **24** (supplement 3), S13–S20.

Moureau, N., Thompson McKinnon, B. & Douglas, C.M. (1999) Multidisciplinary management of thrombotic catheter occlusions in vascular access devices. *Journal of Vascular Access Devices*, **4** (2), 22–29.

National Institute for Clinical Excellence (NICE) (2003) *Infection Control Prevention of Healthcare-associated Infection in Primary and Community Care*, Clinical Guidelines 2. Department of Health, London.

Oncology Nursing Society (1999) *Cancer Chemotherapy Guidelines and Recommendations for Practice*. Oncology Nursing Press, Pittsburgh.

Parker, L. (2002) Management of intravascular devices to prevent infection. *British Journal of Nursing*, **11** (4), 240–246.

Pellowe, C.M., Pratt, R.J., Loveday, H.P., Harper, P., Robinson, N. & Jones, S.R.L.J. (2004) The *epic* project. Updating the evidence base for national evidence based guidelines for preventing healthcare-associated infection in NHS hospitals in England: a report with recommendations. *British Journal of Infection Control*, **5** (6), 10–16.

Perdue, M.B. (2001) Intravenous complications. In: Carlson, K., Perdue, M.B. & Hankins, J. (eds) *Infusion Therapy in Clinical Practice*, 2nd edn. W.B. Saunders, Pennsylvania.

Ponec, D., Irwin, D., Haire, W.D., Hill, P.A., Xin, L. & McClusky, E.R. (2001) Recombinent tissue plasminogen activator (alteplase) for restoration of flow in occluded central venous access devices: a double blind placebo controlled trial – the cardiovascular thrombolytic to open occluded lines (COOL) efficacy trial. *Journal of Vascular and Interventional Radiology*, **12** (8), 951–955.

Pratt, R. (2001) Preventing infections associated with central venous catheters. *Nursing Times*, **97** (15), 36–39.

Raad, I., Dairouche, R., Dupius, J., Abi-Said, D., Gabrielli, A., Hachem, R., Wall, M., Harris, R., Jones, J., Buzard, A., Robertson, C., Sherieq, S., Curling, P., Burke, T., Ericson, L. & Texas Medical Center Study Group (1997) Central venous catheters coated with minocycline and rifampin for the prevention of catheter related colonisation and bloodstream infections. *Annals of Internal Medicine*, **127** (4), 267–274.

Raad, I., Dairouche, R., Hachem, R., Abi-Said, D., Safar, H., Darnwe, T., Mansouri, M. & Morck, D. (1998) Antimicrobial durability and rare ultrastructural colonisation of indwelling central catheters coated with minocycline and rifampin. *Critical Care Medicine*, **26** (2), 219–224.

Ray, C.E. (1999) Infection control principles and practices in the care and management of central venous access devices. *Journal of Intravenous Nursing*, **22** (65), S18–S25.

Reed, T. & Philips, S. (1996) Management of central venous catheters occlusion and repairs. *Journal of Intravenous Nursing*, **19**, 289–294.

Richard Alexander, H. (1994) Clinical performance of long-term venous access devices. In: Richard Alexander, H. (ed.) *Vascular Access In The Cancer Patient: Devices, Insertion Techniques, Maintenance and Prevention and Management of Complications*, pp. 18–36. J.B. Lippincott, Philadelphia.

Rickard, C.M., Courtney, M. & Webster, J. (2004) A survey of ICU practices. *Journal of Central Venous Catheters*, **48** (3, Jan.), 247–256.

Royal College of Nursing (2001) *Administering Intravenous Therapy to Children in the Community Setting: Guidance for Nursing Staff.* Royal College of Nursing, London.

Royal College of Nursing Intravenous Therapy Forum (2003) *Standards for Infusion Therapy.* Royal College of Nursing, London.

Ryder, M. (2001) The role of biofilm in vascular catheter related infections. *New Developments in Vascular Diseases*, **2** (2), 15–21.

Rudolph, R. & Larson, D.L. (1987) Aetiology and treatment of chemotherapeutic agent extravasation injuries: a review. *Journal of Clinical Oncolgy*, **5** (7), 1116–1126.

Schulmeister, L. (1989) Needle dislodgement from implanted venous access devices – inpatient and outpatient experiences. *Journal of Intravenous Nursing*, **12**, 90–92.

Schulmeister, L. (1998) A complication of vascular access device insertion. *Journal of Intravenous Nursing*, **21** (4), 197–202.

Schulmeister, L. & Camp Sorrell, D. (2000) Chemotherapy extravasation from implanted ports. *Oncology Nursing Forum*, **27** (3), 531–560.

Simcock, L. (2001) Use of central venous catheters. *Nursing Times*, **97** (18), 34–35.

Stanley, A. (2002) Managing complications of chemotherapy administration. In: Allwood, M. (ed.) *The Cytotoxic Handbook*, 4th edn. Radcliffe Medical Press, Oxford.

Tebbs, S.E., Trend, V. & Elliott, T.S.J. (1995) The potential reduction of microbial contamination of central venous catheters. *Journal of Hospital Infection*, **30**, 107–113.

Timoney, J.P., Malkin, M.G., Leone, D.M., Groeger, J.S., Heaney, M.L., Keefe, D.L., Klang, M., Lucarelli, C.D., Muller, R.J., Eng, S.L., Connor, M., Small, T.N., Brown, A.E. & Saltz, L.B. (2002) Safe and effective use of alteplase for the clearance of occluded central venous access devices. *Journal of Clinical Oncology*, **20** (7), 1918–1922.

Verhage, A.H. & van Bommel, E.F.H. (1999) Catheter fracture: an under-recognised and serious condition. *Journal of Vascular Access Devices*, **4** (2, Summer), 33–34.

Vesely, T.M. (2003) Central venous catheter tip position: a continuing controversy. *Journal of Cardiovascular and Interventional Radiology*, **14** (5), 527–534.

Weinstein, S.M. (2001) *Plumer's Principles and Practice of Infusion Therapy*, 7th edn, Lippincott Williams & Wilkins, Philadelphia.

Wickham, R., Purl, S. & Welker, D. (1992) Long-term central venous catheters: issues for care. *Seminars in Oncology Nursing*, **8** (2), 133–147.

Wilson, J. (2001) Preventing infection associated with intravenous therapy. In: Wilson, J. (ed.) *Infection Control in Clinical Practice*, 2nd edn. Bailliere Tindall, London.

Young, A.M., Begum, G., Billingham, L.J., Hughes, A.I., Kerr, D.J. Rea, D., Stanley, A., Sweeney, A., Wheatley, K., Wilde, J. and WARP Collaborative Group, UK (2005) WARP: a multi-centre prospective randomised controlled trial (RCT) of thrombosis prophylaxis with warfarin in cancer patients with central venous catheters (CVCs). *ASCO Meeting Abstracts*, **1 June**, 8004.

9 | Patient perspective

A central venous access device can be a lifeline for those who require it for long-term access, or it can be a short-term device that is distressing, but a 'means to an end'. Whatever its intended use, patients need to have information and be involved in the selection and care of the device.

LEARNING OBJECTIVES
By the end of this chapter the reader will be able to:

(1) Understand the issues related to living with a CVAD.
(2) Describe how each CVAD can impact on a patient's life.
(3) Discuss the educational needs of patients in relation to their CVAD.
(4) Develop some patient educational materials and training aids.

PATIENTS' VIEWS OF CVADs
A central venous access device can mean different things to different people, depending on the reason it needs to be inserted. For those who are in critical care after surgery it can be a frightening experience for the patient and distressing for the relatives, but for the patient who requires chemotherapy it may be a lifeline. How the device is perceived and how the patient complies with care will depend on the patient's involvement in the decision-making process and choice of device. Patients who have long-term access devices inserted are now more involved in not only the type of device, but also the finer details of the device, for example with a port: the size, weight, profile and position within the body. Manufacturers involve patients and get feedback on devices in order to improve the design and usability.

Matheny (2002), who is a nurse and has lived with a long-term CVAD, wrote that one of the hardest parts of having a CVAD was taking care of it day after day, that she was extremely overcautious with the sterile technique and was very protective of her device, especially when it became apparent that other nurses did not take care as seriously. Other patients have highlighted that the catheter is their lifeline, in that they will need it for the rest of their life, and as sites become limited they become more anxious when people do not take care (Oley Foundation 2002). Thompson et al. (1997) found that patients who had external catheters listed problems related to the device, such as bulkiness of the clamps (an issue resolved by the advent of valved catheters), exit site position making it difficult to wear a seat belt, and issues related to the scars left following removal. Daniels (1995b) also raised other issues related to long-term CVADs, which included body image, sexuality and change to normal activities.

In a study, Chernecky (2001) examined patients' satisfaction and dissatisfaction with implanted ports in an outpatient oncology setting. She found that more than 50% had had previous problems with intravenous cannulations and venepuncture, with patients reporting that they were extremely happy with their ports. The three main benefits were:

(1) decreased pain compared with cannulation;
(2) the need for fewer needle insertions;
(3) quicker blood sampling.

The negative experiences were infrequent, but 29% of subjects cited monthly heparinisation, sleep disturbances and site soreness following chemotherapy treatment. Overall, 92% stated that the port had improved their quality of life. Other positive comments were that it enabled quick access for emergency treatment, had low maintenance and reduced the emotional stress of receiving chemotherapy. The recommendation from the study was for nurses to assess and recommend a long-term VAD to patients receiving multiple chemotherapy treatments at an earlier stage.

There was a problem with refusal by non-oncology personnel to use the port for intravenous access. This is a common problem and can be seen from both the patients' and staff's perspective:

(1) Why insert a needle and/or have difficulty when the patient has a viable access device in situ?
(2) However, should a nurse who has no knowledge and/or skills be attempting to use a CVAD when they could cause potential problems for the patient by not managing the device appropriately?

There was also a psychological effect of having something foreign left in the body. Sometimes the device would not enable adequate bloods to be taken for a blood test and this was frustrating for patients.

Body image

A CVAD may affect body image in a number of ways (Daniels 1995a):

(1) Due to the physical presence there could be an alteration of body appearance and a feeling of invasion of the body integrity.
(2) It may influence types of clothes worn.
(3) It may interfere with bodily expression of closeness and sexuality.
(4) It may also act as a reminder of the diagnosis and need for treatment.
(5) Its presence can have implications on how others view the role and function of the individual.
(6) It may even 'disable' the individual psychologically if not physically.

In a study, Mirro et al. (1989) compared body image in patients with external catheters versus those with an implanted port. They found that body image was less of a problem when patients had a port in situ. However, this was altered when patients had a port in a position that made it more obvious externally. In those patients the impact on their body image was similar to those who had an external catheter, proving that position of the device has an impact on body image (Mirro et al. 1989). Bow et al. (1999) examined safety, efficacy and the impact on the quality of life of patients with a vascular access port during chemo-therapy and found they had no detectable impact on the func-tional quality of life, although there was less access-related anxiety, pain and discomfort.

Sexuality and body image are affected by cancer, including the intrusion of intravenous devices (Price 1992). The RCN (1992) noted that long-term CVC access could constantly remind the patient of their disease status. In a small study by Oakley et al. (2000) interviews were carried out with patients to ascertain their perceptions of PICCs. Day-to-day living/adapting were discussed and patients adjusted well and were often satisfied with the device. One commented, 'I can hardly feel any differ-ence from that arm to that arm it is very comfortable' (Oakley et al. 2000, page 212). Only one patient referred to an alteration in her body image and found it distressing when other people enquired about the catheter. Social attitudes had an impact on perceived body image for two patients. Restriction to work was linked to devices, but sometimes was a combination of the device and treatment (e.g. chemotherapy via a pump) as well as an illness (such as cancer).

Adaptation was required for sleeping and clothing, as well as bathing, which some found disruptive. Patients also voiced concern in protecting their device, especially when bathing, sleeping and performing manual work, or when dealing with small children. But it rarely seemed to restrict arm movement and the benefit overrode any inconvenience. Nurses asked about alteration in body image commented that PICCs resulted in less alteration than a skin-tunnelled catheter as they were less intrusive and easier to conceal (although this may not be so easy in summer), but PICCs were perceived as more fragile.

Gabriel (2000) also examined patients requiring a PICC for antibiotics, chemotherapy and blood products, their views of PICCs and their individual perceptions on the effect the PICC had on their life, as opposed to those arising from their under-lying medical condition. Half of the patients had had previous experiences of other types of CVADs (five tunnelled, one port). One patient stated that her PICC prevented her from soaking in the bath, but there were no other negative responses. Most reported that they had become accustomed to the PICC being in their arm and were not prevented from doing anything they would normally do. All commented on how easy, comfortable and painless the PICC was when inserted and removed, and felt it had made treatment easier for them.

Daniels (1995b) reported that 19 out of 21 patients with skin-tunnelled catheters felt it had had some degree of impact on their dress in that there was a problem of having to keep the device covered and wearing baggy clothes. Some patients expressed the view that they were either not affected by the device or it was just another facet of their illness. Some talked about wanting to hide it, especially from children and two patients referred to the scar it left after removal. Some had found it difficult to show to their partners and felt that it had affected their sexual relationship. Other problems included being unable to participate in sports and other activities, and difficulties with bathing and sleep positioning due to the catheter. Overall, however, patients found the CVAD advantageous in terms of its convenience and reduced requirement for peripheral venepuncture.

The detriment to physical appearance and body image can be minimised by careful placement of the device. Speechley & Davidson (1989) suggest that a port should be sited away from skin folds and breast tissue for reasons of access. This approach to siting could be applied for cosmetic reasons related to body image, such as avoiding the sternal area, using the less dominant side so it interferes less with arm movement, but recognising that positioning is dependent on the patient's anatomy and disease (Daniels 1995a).

Change to normal activities

This can be related to everyday activities such as bathing, or sporting activities such as swimming. Patients often find that the difficulties in carrying out normal activities, such as bathing, can be a problem. This is particularly true if the device is attached to a pump. One of the issues related to long-term CVADs is that of not being able to swim. Patients are usually advised not to swim because of the concern that swimming may increase the risk of catheter related infections. This aspect was examined in more detail by Robbins et al. (2000) in relation to children with long-term CVCs and the effect on their quality of life of not being able to swim. The study findings demonstrated that in the data generated (using a questionnaire completed by parents on the swimming habits of their children), there was no higher incidence of catheter-related infection in children who swam when compared with those who did not swim. Despite some limitations of the study it resulted in a change of their policy to allow swimming.

Patients' preferences related to CVADs

When patients have had the opportunity to experience a number of devices they can highlight the good and bad points of living with the device, such as how easy it was to use and care for and the degree of problems associated with it. These will influence how they feel about their device. For example, a patient who had previously had two tunnelled catheters, which were both removed due to infection, preferred her PICC, which lasted six months without problems. The patient who had a port inserted which turned on its side and caused problems every time she had it accessed, ended up wishing she had never had a port inserted, stating it was more trouble that it was worth. Chernecky et al. (2002) found that 92% of patients felt that ports improved their quality of life and 47% wished they had received their port earlier in their disease.

EDUCATION AND TRAINING

Education should take place before a choice is made, prior to the insertion of the device, and then after insertion, with ongoing support. Education should be in the form of verbal discussion supported by written information. These should be at an appropriate level, and the factors influencing learning, such as patient's age, language, physical and emotional status, educational level and current stress levels must be considered (McDermott 1995; Weinstein 2001). This should include the purpose and rationale of CVAD placement and procedures required for care and management, the responsibilities of patients and/or carer and healthcare professionals, an explanation of the routine risks and possible complications (McDermott 1995; Weinstein 2001). A practical demonstration is vital, with the patient given time to have hands on practice under supervision when first using the device, and again support and supervision when at home, until the patient and/or carer feels confident and competent.

It is recommended by RCN (2003) that patients receive instruction and education on the following:

- The vascular access device; prescribed infusion therapy, infection control and care plan (Redman 1997; NICE 2003).
- The potential complications associated with the device and any treatment or therapy (Dougherty 2004).
- The nurse must document the information given and the patient's and/or carer's response in the patient's medical and nursing notes (Redman 1997). Education and training of patients, or caregivers, should be in accordance with the *Code of Professional Conduct* (NMC 2004) and *Guidelines for the Administration of Medicines* (NMC 2002).
- The patient/caregiver should be assessed for ability and willingness to undertake administration of intravenous therapy (Birmingham 1997; Chrystal 1997; Hammond 1998; Cole 1999; Kayley 1999; Stover 2000; RCN 2001) and should be informed in clear and appropriate terminology of all aspects of the therapy, including physical and psychological effects, side effects, risks and benefits (Kayley 1999; INS 2000; NICE 2003).
- Patients should receive a demonstration of care, and verbal and written instructions that are individualised to their cognitive, psychomotor, and behavioural abilities (Redman 1997; Hamilton & Fermo 1998; INS 2000; RCN 2001; NICE 2003) and demonstrate an understanding and ability to perform procedures and care.
- Education, training and written information should be provided that includes the safe storage of the drug and equipment, aseptic technique and handwashing, preparation and administration of the drug and infusion delivery equipment, care and maintenance of the venous access device, side

effects of therapy, spillage precautions, and management and recognition of allergic/anaphylactic reactions (Birmingham 1997; Chrystal 1997; Hammond 1998; Cole 1999; Kayley 1999; Stover 2000; RCN 2001; NICE 2003).

PATIENT INFORMATION SHEETS

There are booklets available for patients, explaining the advantages and disadvantages of CVADs (see Fig. 9.1). The following boxes provide examples of how information can be worded to ensure ease of reading and understanding for patients, and covers some of the common questions related to CVADs. Diagrams are also very important and should be clearly labelled and linked to the text. Size and style of font is important as well as layout.

What is an implanted port?

An implanted port is a device which is inserted under the skin into your body. The usual position is on the chest. The port is made up of a portal body and this is connected via a thin tube (catheter) inserted into one of the body's veins: see diagram below. The port can be felt through the skin. Entry is gained by puncturing the silicone membrane with a special type of needle, which is attached to a length of tubing (an extension set). This enables you to receive fluids and drugs, or have blood samples taken from it. Puncturing the port is similar to pricking the skin with a pin. Naturally, it takes some getting used to, but if it is painful, we can apply local anaesthetic gel to the area 30 minutes before we insert the needle, which will numb the skin.

How is a PICC inserted?

A nurse or doctor will apply a local anaesthetic cream about 30–60 minutes before insertion. This will remove the sensation from the skin over the vein. An introducer needle is inserted into the vein and the catheter is threaded through the needle until the tip is in the correct position. The needle is then removed and only the catheter is left. Sterile tape, a dressing and some extra padding are placed over the catheter to hold it in place and reduce any bleeding which may occur in the first 24 hours. You should avoid excessive arm movement for a few hours after insertion.

Are there any risks involved in insertion of a CVAD?

Occasionally, there can be complications when inserting a catheter, for example the needle or guidewire can scratch the top of your lung, causing a pneumothorax (an air pocket). You would probably be unaware of this, but you may become slightly breathless. A pneumothorax would show up on X-ray and would be treated straight away. The catheter may also not thread into the correct position. A chest X-ray is taken after the catheter has been inserted to check that it is correctly positioned and also to check that there is no pneumothorax. Sometimes there may be bruising at the site where the needle went into your vein.

SUPPORT FOR PATIENTS ONCE AT HOME

Most patients will be discharged home and care for the CVAD themselves, or care will be undertaken by their carer or a district nurse. Early referral to the district nurse is vital so that adequate support is set up for the patient once at home (Dougherty 2004).

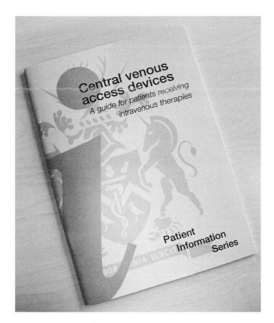

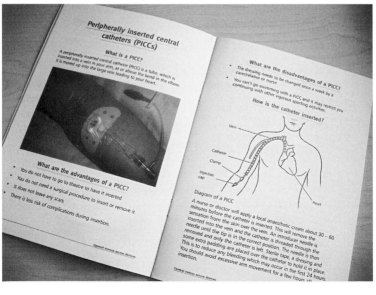

Fig. 9.1 Example pages from a patient information booklet.

A poem by Betty Munnoch
How I came to love my Hickman line

I have a friend
and call him George
fighting my errant calls
along with me.

It was needles here, and needles there
and bruises nearly everywhere,
when a beguiling voice enquired,
Care to try our Hickman line?
Just a little plastic tube winding
its way along your vein.

Strange burrowing snake
making a home on the chest?
My chest?

Emerging with dapper plastic nodes
in Afro mode, bright red and blue, flopping
freely on the breast.
Ready for a topless dance or
to transmit a measured poison.
Mini-Med marvel
of our age
worn discreetly at the waist.

Treatment at home the lure,
and I was caught,
admitting a new partner
to my life and bed.

I feared to harm him in my restless sleep.
But he ticks beside me patiently all night,
only aroused to gentle buzzing
by heavy pressure on his plastic line.

(Reproduced from Munnoch 2001 with permission)

Scenario

Miss Sparks, an 18-year-old woman with cystic fibrosis, has been told that she will need to have a central venous access device as her peripheral veins are now becoming too difficult to access and she is requiring antibiotics on a more frequent basis. She has heard various negative stories from fellow patients about ports and tunnelled catheters and she is really unsure what is best.

What can you do to help her decide what device to choose?

First, one should ascertain what she has heard about the devices and ensure that she has all the correct facts. Show her the different devices and where they would be located, and give her written information sheets and diagrams so she can read it all at her leisure and show and involve her parents. Give her contact details so she can phone and ask any questions and let her speak to patients with positive stories on each type of device so that she has a balanced view.

CONCLUSION

It is vital that patients are well informed and able to be involved in the decision-making process. They are the ones living with the device, whether it is for two weeks or ten years. Involvement promotes a feeling of control, better compliance with care and improved quality of life.

REFERENCES

Birmingham, J. (1997) Decision matrix for selection of patients for a home infusion therapy program. *Journal of Intravenous Nursing*, **20** (5), 258–263.

Bow, E.J., Kilpatrick, M.G. & Clinch, J.J. (1999) Totally implantable venous access ports system for patients receiving chemotherapy for solid-tissue malignancies: a randomised controlled clinical trial examining the safety, efficacy, costs and impact on quality of life. *Journal of Clinical Oncology*, **17** (4), 1267.

Chernecky, C. (2001) Satisfaction versus dissatisfaction with venous access devices in outpatient oncology: a pilot study. *Oncology Nursing Forum*, **28** (10), 1613–1616.

Chernecky, C., Macklin, D., Nugent, K. & Warner, J.L. (2002) The need for shared decision making in the selection of VADs: an assessment of patient and clinicians. *Journal of Vascular Access Devices*, **7** (3), 34–39.

Chrystal, C. (1997) Administering continuous vesicant chemotherapy in the ambulatory setting. *Journal of Intravenous Nursing*, **20** (2), 78–88.

Cole, D. (1999) Selection and management of central venous access devices in the home setting. *Journal of Intravenous Nursing*, **22** (6), 315–319.

Daniels, L.E. (1995a) The physical and psychological implications of central venous access in cancer patients – a review of the literature. *Journal of Cancer Care*, (4), 141–145.

Daniels, L.E. (1995b) Exploring the physical and psychological implications of central venous access in cancer patients – interviews with patients. *Journal of Cancer Care*, (5), 45–48.

Dougherty, L. (2004) Vascular access devices. In: Dougherty, L. & Lister, S. (eds) *Manual of Clinical Nursing Procedures*, 6th edn. Blackwell Science, Oxford.

Gabriel, J. (2000) What patients think of PICC. *Journal of Vascular Access Devices*, **5** (4), 26–30.

Hamilton, H. & Fermo, K. (1998) Assessment of patients requiring intravenous therapy via a central venous route. *British Journal of Nursing*, **7** (8), 451–460.

Hammond, D. (1998) Home intravenous antibiotics: the safety factor. *Journal of Intravenous Nursing*, **21** (2), 81–95.

Intravenous Nursing Society (INS) (2000) *Standards for Infusion Therapy*, Beckon Dickinson and Intravenous Nursing Society, Massachusetts, USA.

Kayley, J. (1999) Intravenous therapy in the community. In: Dougherty, L. & Lamb, J. (eds) *Intravenous Therapy in Nursing Practice*. Churchill Livingstone, Edinburgh.

McDermott, M.K. (1995) Patient education and compliance issues associated with access devices. *Seminars in Oncology Nursing*, **11** (3), 221–226.

Matheny, M. (2002) Teaching patients and nurses from a unique perspective on living with TPN. *Journal of Vascular Access Devices*, **7** (3), 46–48.

Mirro, J., Rao, B.N., Stokes, D.C. & Austin, B.A. (1989) A prospective study of Hickman/Broviac catheters and implantable ports in paediatric oncology patients. *Journal of Clinical Oncology*, **7**, 214–222.

Munnoch, B. (2001) How I came to love my Hickman line. *European Journal of Oncology Nursing*, **5** (2), 77.

National Institute for Clinical Excellence (NICE) (2003) *Infection Control Prevention of Healthcare Associated Infection in Primary and Community Care*, Clinical Guidelines 2. Department of Health, London.

Nursing and Midwifery Council (NMC) (2002) *Guidelines for the Administration of Medicines*. Nursing and Midwifery Council, London.

Nursing and Midwifery Council (NMC) (2004) *Code of Professional Conduct*, Nursing and Midwifery Council, London.

Oakley, C., Wright, E. & Ream, E. (2000) The experiences of patients and nurses with a nurse-led peripherally inserted central venous catheter line service. *European Journal of Cancer*, **4** (4), 207–218.

Oley Foundation (2002) Vascular access devices from a consumer's perspective. Oley Patient Panel. Presented at National Association of Vascular Access Networks 15th International Conference (January). Alexandria, Virginia.

Price, B. (1992) Living with altered body image: the cancer experience. *British Journal of Nursing*, **1** (3), 641–645.

Redman, B.K. (1997) Evaluation and research in patient education. In: Redman, B.K. (ed.) *The Practice of Patient Education*, 8th edn. Mosby, St Louis.

Robbins, J., Cromwell, P. & Korones, D.N. (2000) Swimming and central venous catheter-related infections in children with cancer. In: Nolan, M.T. & Mock, V. (eds) *Measuring Patient Outcomes*, pp. 169–184. Sage Publications, London.

Royal College of Nursing (1992) *Guidelines for the Management of Skin-tunnelled Catheters*. Royal College of Nursing, London.

Royal College of Nursing (2001) *Administering Intravenous Therapy to Children in the Community Setting: Guidance for Nursing Staff*. Royal College of Nursing, London.

Royal College of Nursing Intravenous Therapy Forum (2003) *Standards for Infusion Therapy*. Royal College of Nursing, London.

Speechley, V. & Davidson, T. (1989) Managing an implantable drug delivery system. *Professional Nurse*, **4** (6), 284–288.

Stover, B. (2000) Training the client in self-management of haemophilia. *Journal of Intravenous Nursing*, **23** (5), 304–309.

Thompson, A., Kidd, E., McKenzie, M., Parker, A.C. & Nixon, S.J. (1997) Long-term central venous access: the patients' view. *Intensive Therapy Clinical Monitoring*, **10** (5), 142–145.

Wilson, J. (2001) Preventing infection associated with intravenous therapy. In: Wilson, J. (ed.) *Infection Control in Clinical Practice*, 2nd edn. Bailliere Tindall, London.

Weinstein, S.M. (2001) *Plumer's Principles and Practice of Infusion Therapy*, 7th edn, Lippincott Williams & Wilkins, Philadelphia.

Appendix 1
The AccessAbility
Decision-Making Model

The AccessAbility™ is an internet-based decision making model designed to help healthcare professionals select the most appropriate venous access device. AccessAbility™ is a registered trademark of C.R. Bard, Inc.

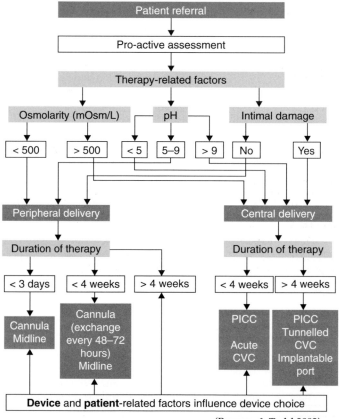

(Bravery & Todd 2002)

Appendix 2
Consent form for PICC insertion

To be retained in patient's notes	Patient's surname/family name
	Patient's first names
	Date of birth
	Responsible health professional
	Job title
	NHS number (or other identifier)
Insertion of a Peripherally Inserted Central Catheter (PICC)	☐ Male ☐ Female
Patient agreement to investigation or treatment	Special requirements (e.g. other language/other communication method)

Name of proposed procedure or course of treatment (including brief explanation if medical term not clear)

Insertion of a peripherally inserted central catheter (PICC)
This catheter is inserted into a vein in your arm and threaded up into the main vein to your heart called superior vena cava. Before insertion, local anaesthetic cream will be applied to the vein to ensure you do not feel any pain during the procedure. This takes about 30 minutes to work. The procedure takes about 30 minutes and then you will be sent for a Chest X-Ray.

STATEMENT OF HEALTH PROFESSIONAL (to be filled in by health professional with appropriate knowledge of proposed procedure, as specified in Consent Policy)

I have explained the proposed procedure to the patient. In particular, I have explained:

- **The intended benefits:**

☐ This catheter will enable you to have a reliable form of venous access in order to receive your therapy.

☐ _____
_____
_____
_____
_____

STATEMENT OF HEALTH PROFESSIONAL (Cont.)

- **Serious or frequently occurring risks:**

☐ There are some risks during insertion – firstly that the needle could cause a bruise or 'haematoma'. The catheter may not thread into the correct position or the guidewire can scratch the top of your lung causing a pneumothorax (an air pocket). You would probably be unaware of this but you may become slightly breathless – both of these complications would be identified on the chest X ray you will have following the insertion procedure and be treated straight away.

Once the catheter is in place there is a risk of infection and also a clot forming around the catheter. You may be given a drug called warfarin (a blood thinning agent) to reduce the risk of this occurring.

Any other risks:
_____
_____

Any extra procedures which may become necessary during the procedure:

☐ blood transfusion

☐ other procedure (please specify)
_____
_____
_____
_____

I have also discussed what the procedure is likely to involve, the benefits and risks of any available alternative treatments (including no treatment) and any particular concerns of this patient.

The following leaflet/tape has been provided:

☐ **Introduction to PICC**

☐ _____

_____

This procedure will involve:

☐ **General and/or regional anaesthesia**   ☐ **Local anaesthesia**

☐ **Sedation**

Signed   **Date:**

Name (Print):   **Job Title:**

Contact details (if patient wishes to discuss options later) _____

_____

_____

_____

_____

STATEMENT OF INTERPRETER (where appropriate)

Language Line ref: _____

I have interpreted the information above to the patient to the best of my ability and in a way in which I believe s/he can understand

Interpreter's signature: **Date:**

Name (Print):

Top copy accepted by patient: Yes / No (Please ring)

Continued

STATEMENT OF PATIENT

Please read this form carefully. If your treatment has been planned in advance, you should already have your own copy which describes the benefits and risks of the proposed treatment. If not, you will be offered a copy now. If you have any further questions, do ask – we are here to help you. You have the right to change your mind at any time, including after you have signed this form.

I agree to the procedure or course of treatment described on this form.

I understand that you cannot give me a guarantee that a particular person will perform the procedure. The person will, however, have appropriate experience.

I understand that I will have the opportunity to discuss the details of anaesthesia with an anaesthetist before the procedure, unless the urgency of my situation prevents this. (This only applies to patients having general or regional anaesthesia.)

I understand that any procedure in addition to those described on this form will only be carried out if it is necessary to save my life or to prevent serious harm to my health.

I have been told about additional procedures which may become necessary during my treatment. I have listed below any procedures **which I do not wish to be carried out** without further discussion

Patient's signature: **Date:**

Name (Print):

A witness should sign below if the patient is unable to sign but has indicated his or her consent. Young people/children may also like a parent to sign here (see notes).

Signature: **Date:**

Name (Print):

CONFIRMATION OF CONSENT (to be completed by a health professional when the patient is admitted for the procedure, if the patient has signed the form in advance)

On behalf of the team treating the patient, I have confirmed with the patient that s/he has no further questions and wishes the procedure to go ahead.

Signed: **Date:**

Name (Print):   **Job Title:**

Important notes: (tick if applicable)

☐ See also advance directive/living will (e.g. Jehovah's Witness form)

☐ Patient has withdrawn consent (ask patient to sign /date here)

Appendix 3
Sources of information

Royal College of Nursing

The Royal College of Nursing Intravenous Therapy Forum was established in 2000 (previously it was known as the RCN Intravenous Special Interest group, but began life as BITA: British Intravenous Therapy Association). The forum is made up of nurses interested in intravenous therapy and vascular access devices and provides a twice yearly newsletter on intravenous issues. It is a source of information and advice and published the *Standards for Infusion Therapy* in October 2003. For information or to join look at www.rcn.org.uk or call RCN direct on 0845 772 6100.

Infusion Nurses Society

Infusion Nurses Society (formerly the Intravenous Nursing Society) is an American organisation that specialises in infusion therapy. Membership entitles the nurse to receive the journal, *Infusion Nursing*, every two months, as well as giving access to a large number of educational materials including the text book *Infusion Therapy in Clinical Practice*, last published in 2001. To join visit www.ins1.org.

Association of Vascular Access

Association of Vascular Access (formerly NAVAN) is also an American organisation devoted to vascular access. Membership entitles the nurse to receive the *Journal of Association of Vascular Access (JAVA)* four times a year. To join visit www.navannet. org.

Booklist

Carlson, K., Perdue, M.B. & Hankins, J. (eds) (2001) *Infusion Therapy in Clinical Practice*, 2nd edn. W.B. Saunders, Pennsylvania.

Dougherty, L. & Lamb, J. (1999) *Intravenous Therapy in Nursing Practice*. Churchill Livingstone, Edinburgh.

Dougherty, L. & Lister, S. (2004) *The Royal Marsden Manual of Clinical Nursing Procedures*, 6th edn. Blackwell Publishing, Oxford.

Finley, T. (2004) *Intravenous Therapy*. Blackwell Publishing, Oxford.

Intravenous Nursing Society (INS) (2000) *Standards for Infusion Therapy*, Beckon Dickinson and Intravenous Nursing Society, Massachusetts, USA.

Macklin, D. & Chernecky, C. (2004) *Intravenous Therapy*. Saunders, St Louis.

McPhee, A. (1999) *Handbook of Infusion Therapy*. Springhouse Corporation, Pennsylvania.

Royal College of Nursing (2003) *RCN Standards for Infusion Therapy*. Royal College of Nursing, London.

Weinstein, S.M. (2001) *Plumer's Principles and Practice of Infusion Therapy*, 7th edn, Lippincott Williams & Wilkins, Philadelphia.

Index

Note: page numbers in *italics* refer to figures, those in **bold** refer to tables. Central venous access devices are referred to as 'CVAD'.